Contents

Preface

Who is this book for?

This book is for people who would like to know more about caring for their bodies. To do this they must know something about how the human body works, in other words, human biology. Not all people like studying detailed anatomical drawings or reading accounts of how the body is made and how it works. However, most people enjoy cartoons, so many of the facts in this book are introduced through cartoon-style drawings, although there is some reading to go with them.

How it is supposed to be used?

Learning things first-hand from experiments and seeing things for yourself is great, but most people need something to help them remember what they actually did in class. Memories soon fade and what we think we remember may not always be right. So, when you have learned about the structure of the gut and have seen a rabbit or rat gut dissected in class, you can apply what you have learned to the human gut and use this book to help you understand what causes diarrhoea and constipation and how to avoid them. Why do those fit and healthy looking guardsmen faint? When you have learned about the circulation of the blood in class, you will be able to find the answer in this book. So use this book to help you apply what you learn in class.

What about revising for examinations?

Yes, indeed, this book is meant to help you pass GCSE human biology examinations. It should help you to find the gaps in your understanding of how the body works, which is what all good revision is about, rather than just trying to remind you of facts.

Health for You

HUMAN BODY CARE
AND MAINTENANCE

The only machine with a built-in self-repairing mechanism!

**Dorothy Dallas, Jane Jenks and
Barbara Patilla**

It's your life – you can't trade it in for a new model!

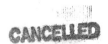
Stanley Thornes (Publishers) Ltd

Originally published in 1987 by Hutchinson Education
Reprinted 1988

Reprinted in 1990 by
Stanley Thornes (Publishers) Ltd
Old Station Drive
Leckhampton
CHELTENHAM GL53 0DN

British Library Cataloguing in Publication Data

Dallas, Dorothy M.
  Health for you.
  1. Health
  I. Title   II. Jenks, Jane   II. Patilla, Barbara
  613   RA776

ISBN 0 7487 0259 8

Typeset in 12 on 13pt VIP Meridien by
DP Media Limited, Hitchin, Hertfordshire
Printed and bound in Great Britain by Martin's of Berwick

1 Food and Energy

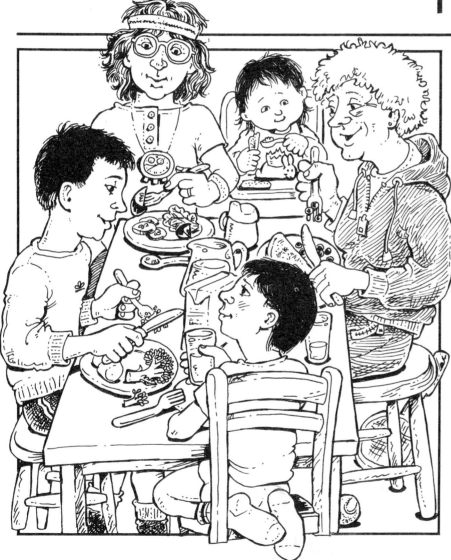

What is food?

Food supplies the fuel and spare parts for your body machine.

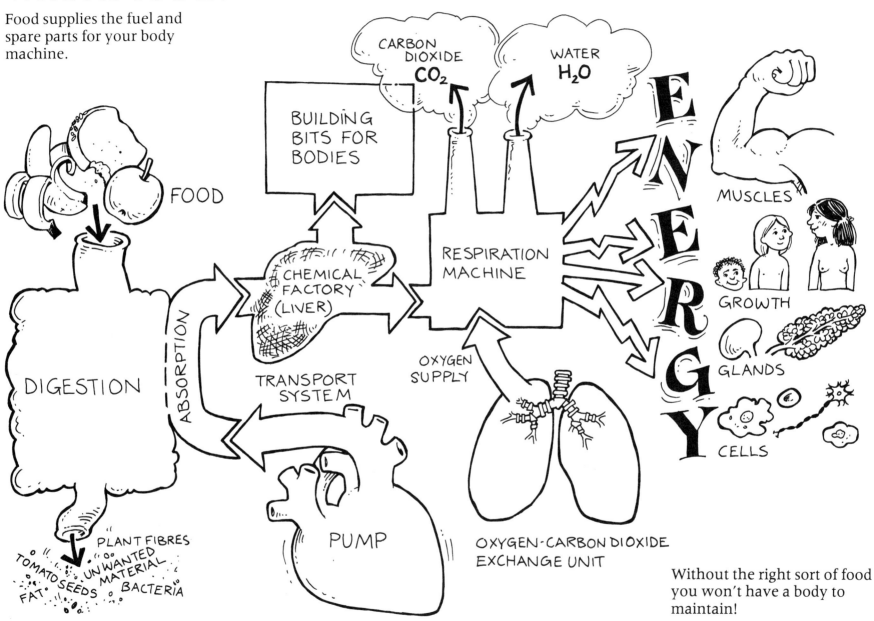

FOOD

CARBON DIOXIDE CO_2

WATER H_2O

BUILDING BITS FOR BODIES

RESPIRATION MACHINE

ENERGY

MUSCLES

GROWTH

GLANDS

CELLS

DIGESTION

ABSORPTION

CHEMICAL FACTORY (LIVER)

TRANSPORT SYSTEM

OXYGEN SUPPLY

PUMP

OXYGEN-CARBON DIOXIDE EXCHANGE UNIT

PLANT FIBRES UNWANTED MATERIAL TOMATO SEEDS BACTERIA FAT

Without the right sort of food you won't have a body to maintain!

What food does

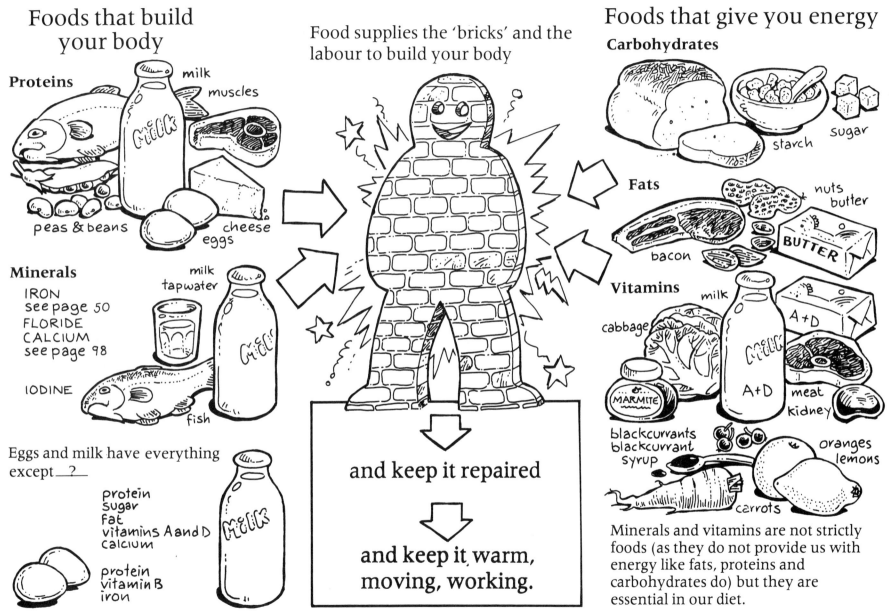

Foods that build your body

Proteins

milk
muscles

peas & beans
cheese
eggs

Minerals

IRON
see page 50
FLORIDE
CALCIUM
see page 98

IODINE

milk
tapwater

fish

Eggs and milk have everything except____?

protein
sugar
fat
vitamins A and D
calcium

protein
vitamin B
iron

Food supplies the 'bricks' and the labour to build your body

and keep it repaired

and keep it warm, moving, working.

Foods that give you energy

Carbohydrates

sugar
starch

Fats

nuts
butter

bacon

BUTTER

Vitamins

milk

cabbage

A + D

MARMITE

A + D

meat
kidney

blackcurrants
blackcurrant
syrup

oranges
lemons

carrots

Minerals and vitamins are not strictly foods (as they do not provide us with energy like fats, proteins and carbohydrates do) but they are essential in our diet.

7

What should you eat?

Don't eat too much

1 Too much protein – strain on your liver.

2 Too much fat – overweight, clogged arteries.

3 Too much cabbage – can stop you absorbing iodine, giving you 'cabbage goitre'.

4 You can't!

5 Too much starch is stored as fat.

Eat every day
something from each of these five sections

1 Pure protein (not mixed up as in sausages or pies).

2 One egg every two days harms no-one. Most people eat too much fried food and pastry.

3 Leafy vegetables (as raw as possible). Cress, cabbage, lettuce, celery, fresh (or frozen) spinach.

4 Fresh fruit Blackcurrants have the most vitamin C in them, next are oranges, lemons, grapefruit.

5 Starch (which is turned into sugar when digested). Peas and beans have protein as well as starch.

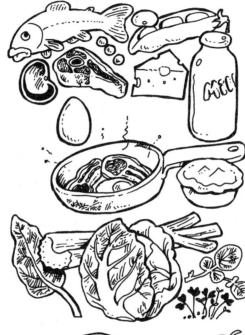

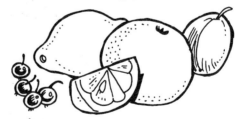

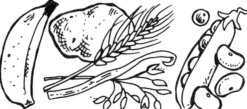

If you don't

a Not enough to repair skin, muscles, etc.

b You miss out on B vitamins and iron and calcium.

a Not enough under your skin to keep you warm.

b You miss out on vitamins A and D.

a Constipation! Vegetable fibres 'sweep out' your 'insides'.

b Minerals and B vitamins too, are missed.

a Vitamin C, the great disease-fighter, is missed.

b Just enough sugar – not enough to rot your teeth.

a It is the main source of energy and if you don't have enough you use up valuable protein instead.

b You will feel 'empty' (although if you don't eat enough fat you will feel empty anyway).

Balancing your diet

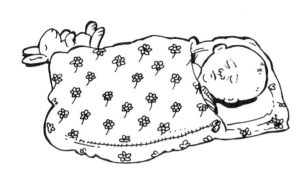

Newborn babies need a lot of water, some body builders and some energy foods. (They are a bit like dried prunes – they need water to expand their cells!)

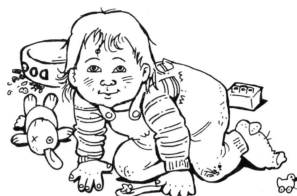

Crawlers obviously need more energy! They can deal with all sorts of food, not just milk.

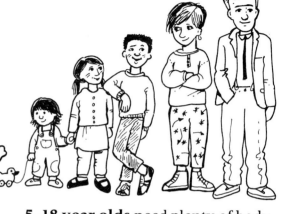

5–18 year olds need plenty of body building 'bricks' – proteins, minerals and vitamins.

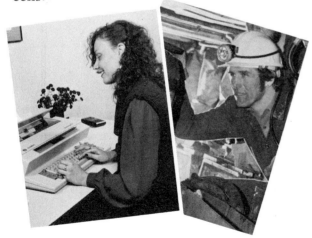

Adults: the food they need depends on the work they do – the more physical exercise, the more fats and carbohydrates.

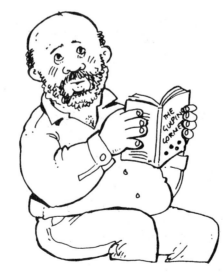

Middle aged: those who move less must eat less!

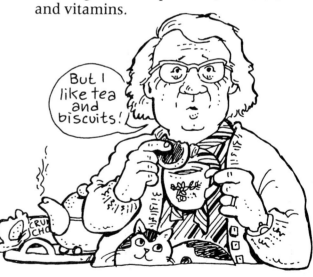

But I like tea and biscuits!

Old people: proteins, vitamins and minerals needed, not just tea and biscuits. Old bodies need to keep well repaired.

Respiration: the release of energy from food

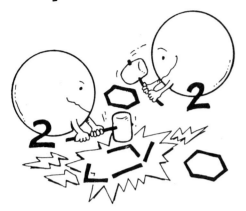

1 Oxygen is needed to break down food and release **energy**.

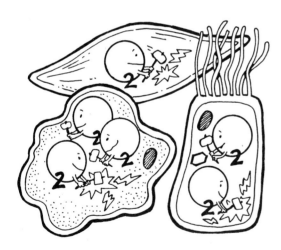

2 This happens in every cell of the body – if it is alive.

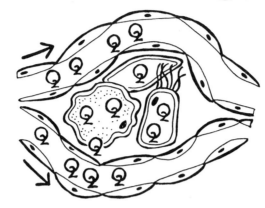

3 So every cell must be near a small blood vessel (capillary) to get oxygen to break down food. These small blood vessels are everywhere – where can you cut yourself without bleeding?

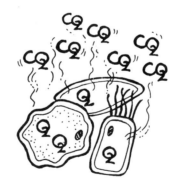

4 And every cell makes lots of carbon dioxide (CO_2) as it uses oxygen to release energy (respires).

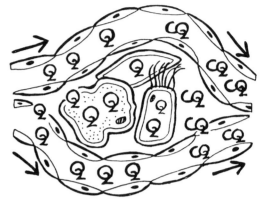

5 But every cell is near a small blood vessel and this takes the carbon dioxide away.

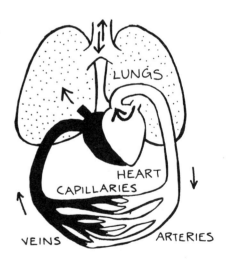

6 So humans need a heart, lungs, arteries, veins and capillaries to take oxygen to the cells and bring carbon dioxide from the cells.

Energy is life

Respiration releases the energy for

Keeping warm, keeping cool

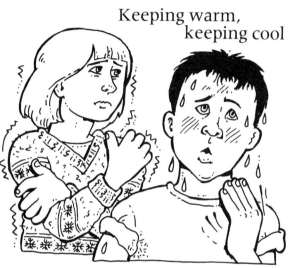

Knowing what goes on

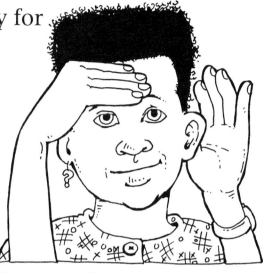

Movement

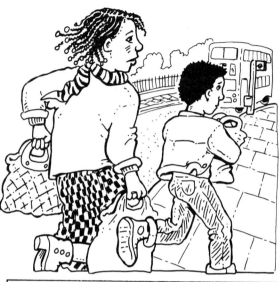

Growth

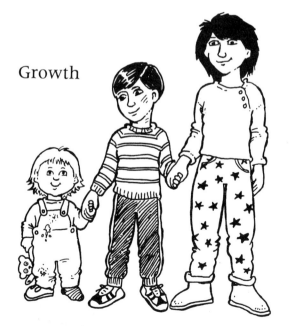

Reproduction

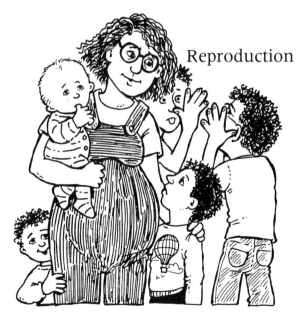

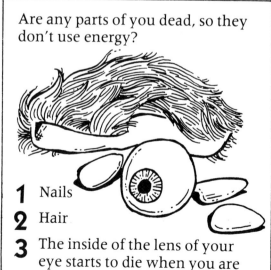

Are any parts of you dead, so they don't use energy?

1 Nails

2 Hair

3 The inside of the lens of your eye starts to die when you are about 14!

Check-up 1 What do you know about food and energy?

1 Write these sentences out and fill in the blanks. Use the words in the box.

hair   respiration   cells
carbon dioxide   growth

Energy is released from food by a process called .... This happens in the .... of your body. .... is a waste product made here at the same time. The energy released can be used for movement, ..., and many other things. Dead parts of your body, like your ...., do not need energy.

2 Look at these foods. Write each one in the box where you think it goes best.

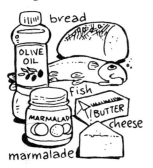

Fat	Protein	Carbohydrate

3 What is meant by a 'high fibre diet'?
Write a few sentences to explain what fibre is and why it is useful in your body.

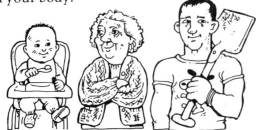

4 Write three sentences for each picture on the type of diet this person needs.

5 Copy this table and fill in the gaps.

What you need in your diet	What it does	Where you can get it
	Gives you energy	Bread
Calcium		Milk
	Builds your body	
Vitamin C		
	Sweeps out your insides	
Fat		

6 Crossword

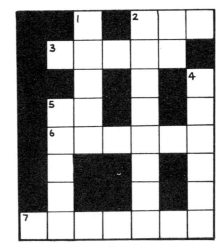

Clues Across
2 Butter contains a lot of this.
3 The place where respiration happens in your body.
5 Are minerals and vitamins really foods?
6 Carbohydrates provide this.
7 You need this food for building up your body.

Clues Down
1 A fruit which contains a lot of vitamin C.
2 This is added to drinking water to strengthen teeth.
4 Joins with carbohydrate in respiration.
5 How often you need to eat sugar.

Your Teeth and Digestive 2 System

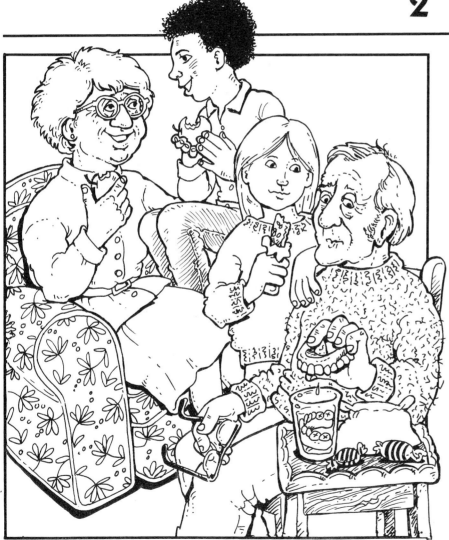

Digestion and indigestion

Much of what you eat is of no use. **Digestion** sorts out the useful from the useless, ready for **absorption** into the blood.

This happens in a tube 1080 cm (10.8 m) long, leading from the mouth to the **anus**.

Anything that can't be smashed up by the teeth and by juices from the **glands** passes out of the anus as **faeces**.

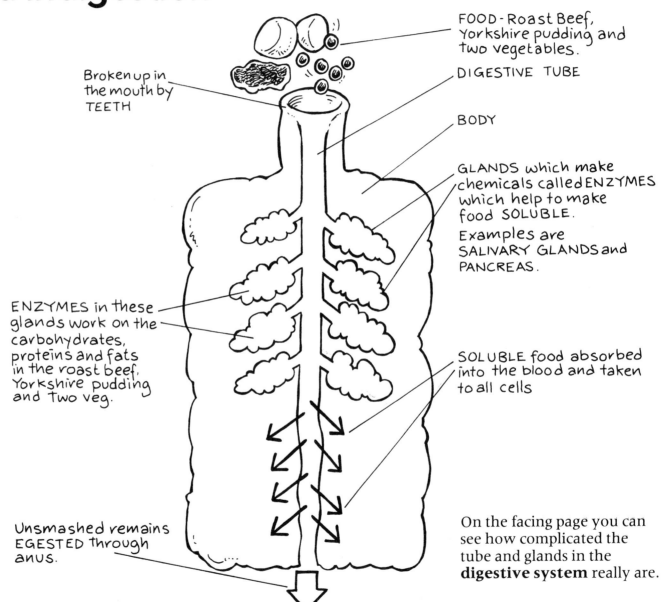

FOOD - Roast Beef, Yorkshire pudding and two vegetables.

Broken up in the mouth by TEETH

DIGESTIVE TUBE

BODY

GLANDS which make chemicals called ENZYMES which help to make food SOLUBLE.
Examples are SALIVARY GLANDS and PANCREAS.

ENZYMES in these glands work on the carbohydrates, proteins and fats in the roast beef, Yorkshire pudding and Two veg.

SOLUBLE food absorbed into the blood and taken to all cells

Unsmashed remains EGESTED through anus.

On the facing page you can see how complicated the tube and glands in the **digestive system** really are.

14

Digestion and indigestion

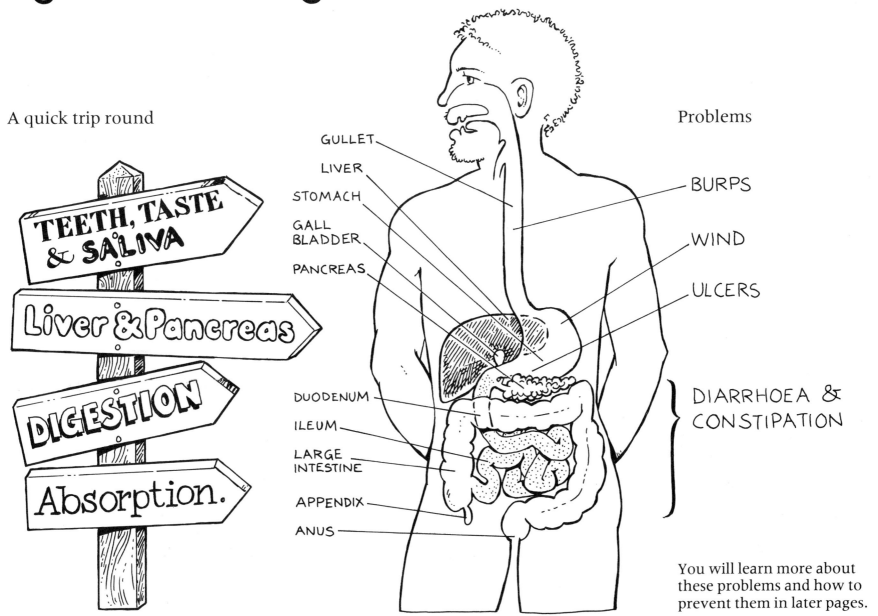

A quick trip round

TEETH, TASTE & SALIVA

Liver & Pancreas

DIGESTION

Absorption.

GULLET
LIVER
STOMACH
GALL BLADDER
PANCREAS
DUODENUM
ILEUM
LARGE INTESTINE
APPENDIX
ANUS

Problems

BURPS

WIND

ULCERS

DIARRHOEA & CONSTIPATION

You will learn more about these problems and how to prevent them in later pages.

False teeth are nice!

They must be, so many people have them!

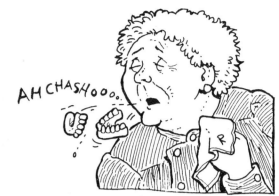

"Who wants real teeth? I can bite into ice cream without my fillings jumping, and dentists don't hurt anymore!"

You sneeze them out – always at the wrong time.

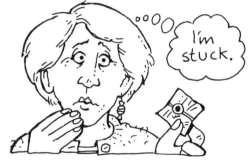

You can't eat toffees or chewing gum – except by yourself.

 If you get fat, they don't fit – they are too tight and you get ulcers.

 If you get thin, they don't fit – they are too loose and they clatter about and may fall out!

 They take time to get used to. You'll whistle while you talk for a week or two.

 You can't eat so quickly!

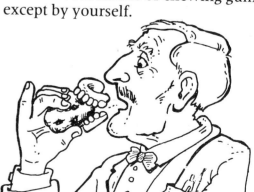

They get attached to soft buns!

How to have good natural teeth

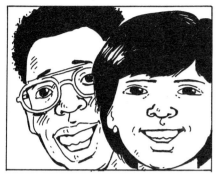

Pick the right parents –
Asian, Caribbean or Chinese
are particularly good.

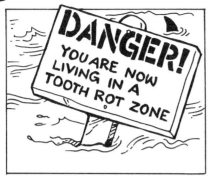

Live in a district which has
fluoride in the drinking
water.

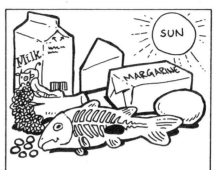

Eat plenty of foods
containing calcium and
vitamin D. Don't eat too
much sweet food.

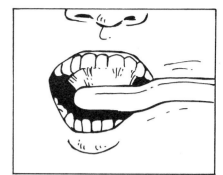

Don't ruin you gums.
Brushing your teeth wrongly
drags your gum away from
your teeth and breaks the
membranes, so germs
(microbes) get in and you
lose another tooth.

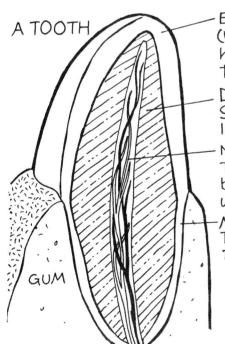

A TOOTH

ENAMEL
(White) Some people don't
have much-they picked
the wrong parents!

DENTINE
Softer than enamel, germs
love it.

NERVES & BLOOD VESSELS
Teeth are alive and need
blood to respire. This is
where it hurts.

MEMBRANE.
This is what keeps the
tooth in it's socket.

GUM

Brush your teeth the right way –always
from gum to tooth.

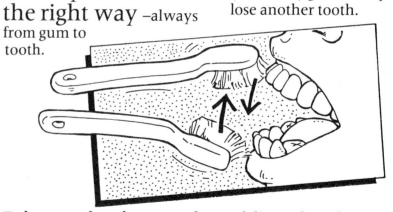

To have good teeth you need a good diet and good
heredity. Everyone knows they *should* clean their teeth
but most people don't. Maybe they like going to the
dentist!
And if you live in an area where there is no fluoride in the
drinking water, brush your teeth with fluoride tooth
paste.

17

How to look after your gums

Toothpicks, wood not metal, stop food packing into spaces between teeth and giving germs (microbes) a home.

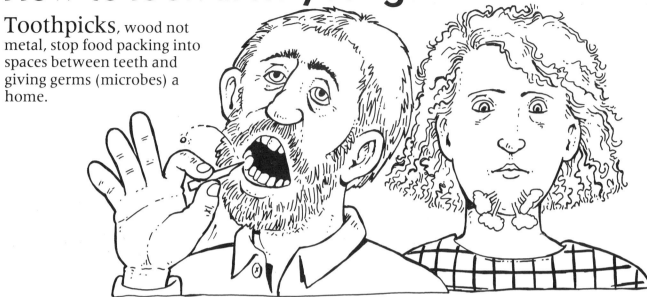

Salivary glands
These swell when you've got mumps.

Saliva rinses gums as well as teeth but a good supply of saliva is inherited. That's why you need the right parents.

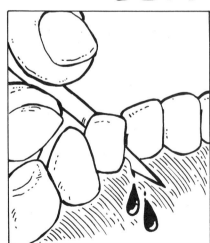

Metal tooth picks cut gums and let germs in.

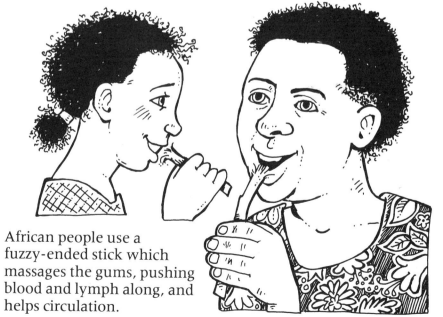

African people use a fuzzy-ended stick which massages the gums, pushing blood and lymph along, and helps circulation.

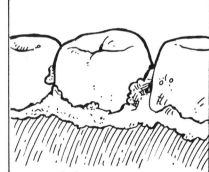

Plaque A mixture of food, saliva and germs that builds up on teeth which aren't brushed enough. Germs stick to it and it pushes your gum away from your tooth leaving room for more germs to get in.

Why false teeth eat more slowly

Natural teeth are

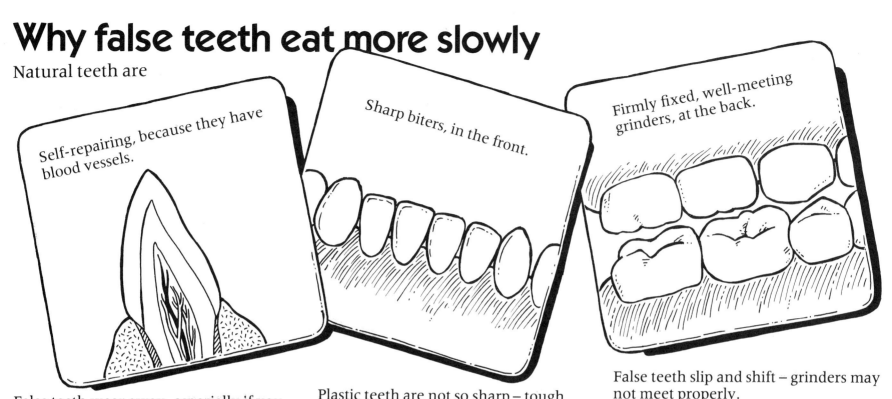

Self-repairing, because they have blood vessels.

Sharp biters, in the front.

Firmly fixed, well-meeting grinders, at the back.

False teeth wear away, especially if you like hard foods like nuts. Your dentist will sharpen them for you if you ask him nicely.

Plastic teeth are not so sharp – tough meat is tough luck for false teeth wearers.

False teeth slip and shift – grinders may not meet properly.

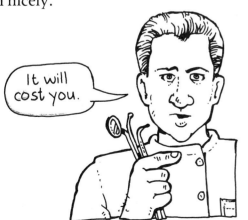

It will cost you.

What are wisdom teeth?

The last grinders to come through, sometimes as late as age 35! Often they are a bad shape and get stuck in the jaw. If they have to come out it's best done in hospital.

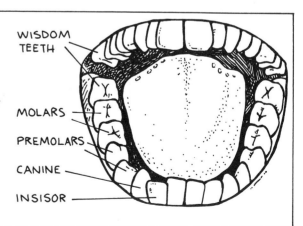

WISDOM TEETH

MOLARS

PREMOLARS

CANINE

INSISOR

What is taste?

What we call taste is really smell plus taste. Food dissolves in your saliva so you can taste it.

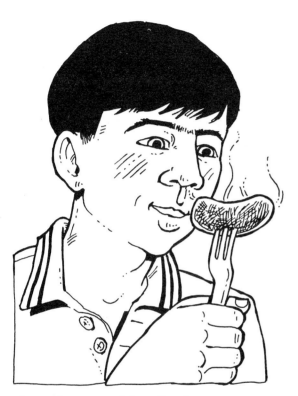

If you have a cold or flu the nerve endings in your nose get covered with extra mucus – so you miss out on 'taste' because you can't smell.

If you haven't tried it, hold your nose, shut your eyes and see if you can tell the difference between a bacon-flavoured and an onion-flavoured potato crisp.

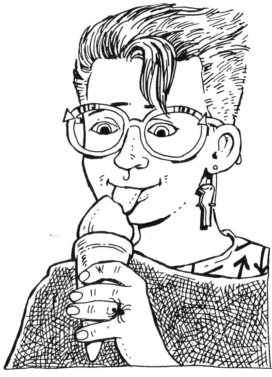

There are taste-detecting nerve endings on your tongue, and there are some in your throat and even on your vocal cords.

Your sort and quantity of saliva (which you inherit from your parents) affects your taste. This is one reason why you might have the same likes and dislikes as your parents.

What use is taste?

Every year children eat poisonous berries like nightshade and privet and the taste didn't put them off. But at least smell tells you when food has gone bad and helps to stop you getting food poisoning.

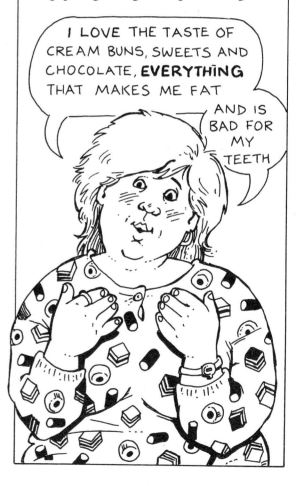

I LOVE THE TASTE OF CREAM BUNS, SWEETS AND CHOCOLATE, **EVERYTHING** THAT MAKES ME FAT

AND IS BAD FOR MY TEETH

What is digestion?

If you look at one of your veins, perhaps one of those on the back of your hand, you don't see the dinner you've just eaten floating through it. So what happens to your food before it gets into your blood?

Chip
Ground up by teeth.
Rolled into a ball by tongue and helped down food tube by saliva.
Drops into your stomach where it is all churned up.

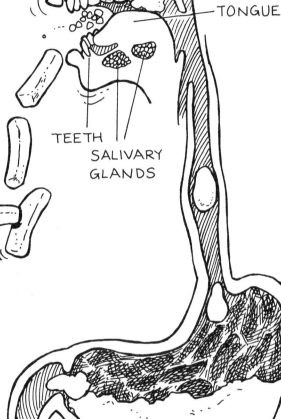

TONGUE

TEETH
SALIVARY
GLANDS

Then each different kind of food has to be smashed up by a different chemical, until it is small enough to get into your blood.

Fat   Some gets broken up.

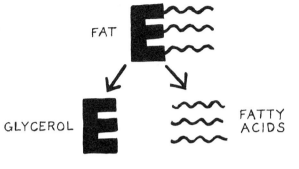

FAT

GLYCEROL

FATTY
ACIDS

Some gets covered with a layer which will dissolve in water and goes into your lymph.

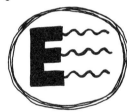

Protein   Muscle (which is what fish and meat really are), eggs, milk, cheese, peas and beans get broken up into very small bits which have many different shapes – **amino acids**.

Carbohydrate   All starches are changed to sugar – usually glucose.

Shape of one molecule of glucose.

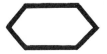

Your liver and gall bladder

Where they are

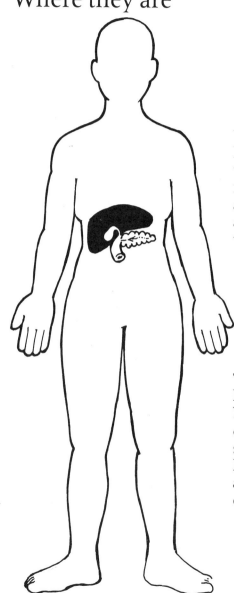

Your liver makes poisons harmless. Alcohol is probably the one it has to cope with most often. Too much alcohol damages your liver and stops it working – giving you cirrhosis of the liver.

The liver makes **bile** which helps dissolve fats. The gall bladder stores bile. Stones can crystallize out of bile and get stuck in your **bile duct**. It hurts every time you eat fat and you may need an operation to get the stone out.

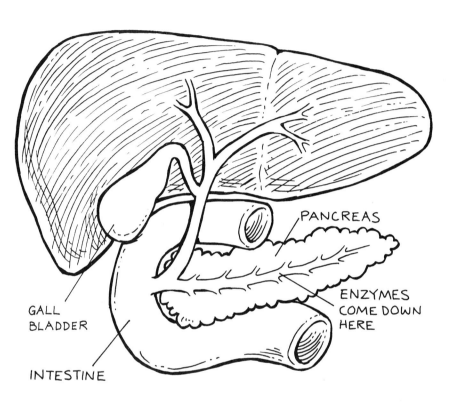

PANCREAS

ENZYMES
COME DOWN
HERE

GALL
BLADDER

INTESTINE

Some other things your liver does

1 Breaks up old protein such as that from red blood cells and uses the bits to make new protein.

2 Packs away glucose as a starch called **glycogen**.

3 Makes **urea**, a waste product, out of protein you no longer need.

22

Your pancreas

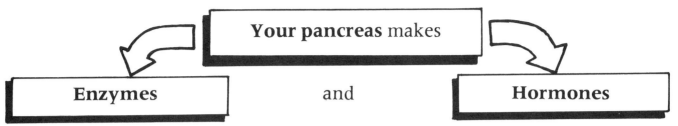

Your pancreas makes

Enzymes and Hormones

the chemicals which smash fats and proteins into molecules of absorbable size.

Examples of hormones are **insulin**, which lowers blood sugar, **glucagon**, which raises it.

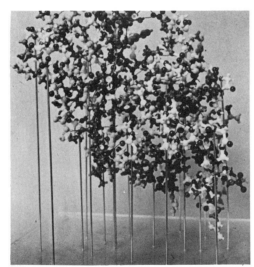

Lysozyme

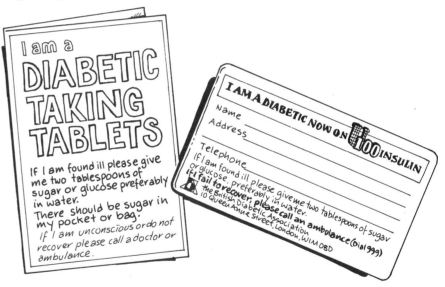

I am a DIABETIC TAKING TABLETS

If I am found ill please give me two tablespoons of sugar or glucose preferably in water.
There should be sugar in my pocket or bag.
If I am unconscious or do not recover please call a doctor or ambulance.

I AM A DIABETIC NOW ON 100 INSULIN

Name
Address

Telephone
If I am found ill please give me two tablespoons of sugar or glucose, preferably in water.
If I fail to recover, please call an ambulance (Dial 999)
the British Diabetic Association
10 Queen Anne Street, London, W1M 0BD

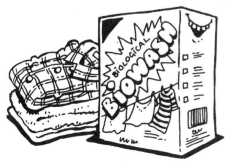

But digestion isn't the only thing enzymes do. For example:
they release C O₂ from blood and energy from glucose and they pack energy into more readily available bits called ATP (see page 87).

Hormones travel in your blood to their targets.

Insulin's target is every cell in the body. It helps glucose get through the cell membrane so the cell can use the energy in the glucose.

Diabetics' sugar stays in their blood, so they can't use the energy in it. They must take insulin or they feel weak and tired.

What are absorption and assimilation?

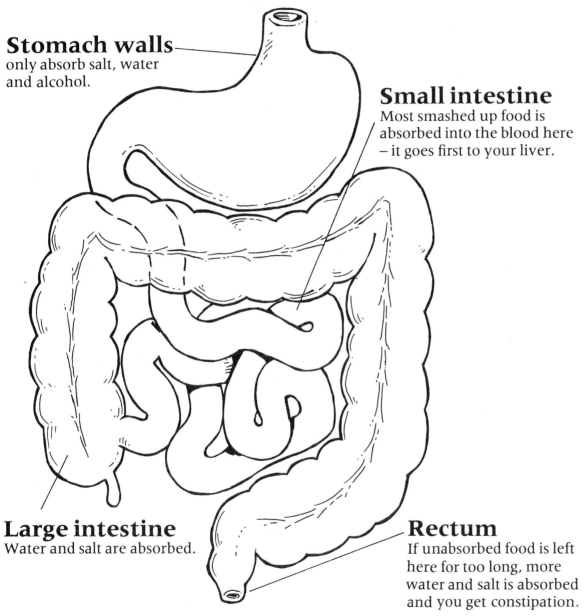

Stomach walls
only absorb salt, water
and alcohol.

Small intestine
Most smashed up food is
absorbed into the blood here
– it goes first to your liver.

Large intestine
Water and salt are absorbed.

Rectum
If unabsorbed food is left
here for too long, more
water and salt is absorbed
and you get constipation.

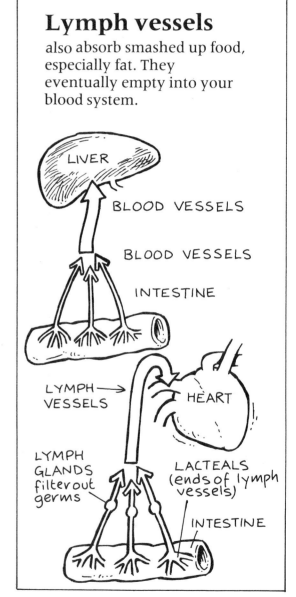

Lymph vessels
also absorb smashed up food,
especially fat. They
eventually empty into your
blood system.

LIVER

BLOOD VESSELS

BLOOD VESSELS

INTESTINE

LYMPH →
VESSELS

HEART

LYMPH
GLANDS
filter out
germs

LACTEALS
(ends of lymph
vessels)

INTESTINE

Why doesn't your food get stuck?

Sometimes it does – don't eat orange peel.

Tummy rumbles – gut walls have muscles which push food and gas or wind.

MUSCLES SQUEEZE BEHIND FOOD

MUSCLES RELAX IN FRONT OF FOOD

Why doesn't milk go straight through?

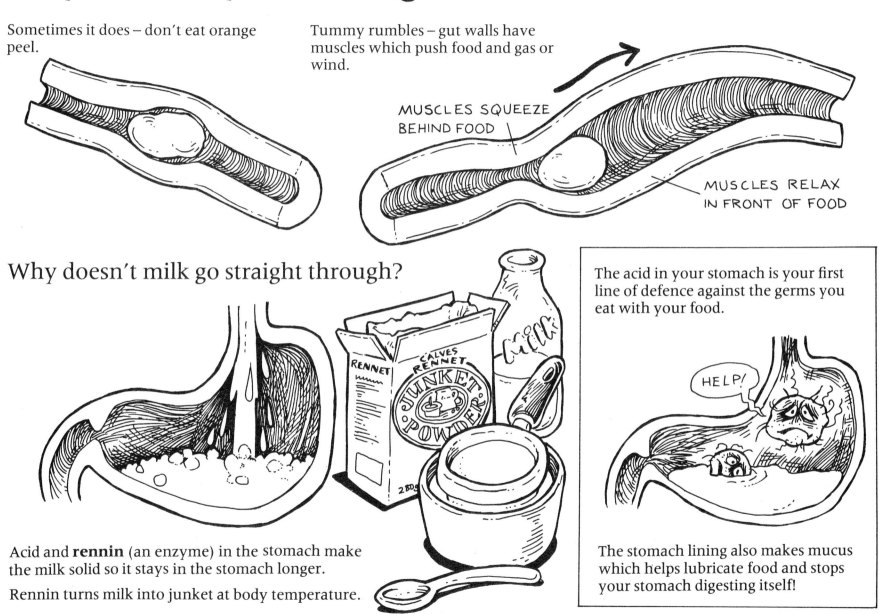

RENNET

CALVES RENNET JUNKET POWDER

280g

MILK

Acid and **rennin** (an enzyme) in the stomach make the milk solid so it stays in the stomach longer.

Rennin turns milk into junket at body temperature.

The acid in your stomach is your first line of defence against the germs you eat with your food.

HELP!

The stomach lining also makes mucus which helps lubricate food and stops your stomach digesting itself!

25

What are vitamins?

Chemicals your body needs, most of which you can't make yourself.

Vitamin A helps you to see, especially in dim light. Found in 'yellow' vegetables like carrots, and in milk, butter, margarine, liver.

Vitamin B (This is really a group of several vitamins called B1, B2 and so on.) Respiration can't work without B vitamins, so you would feel generally tired and unfit without enough of them. Friendly bacteria in your large intestine usually make some B vitamins for you. Antibiotics kill these friendly bacteria as well as the harmful ones, so eat plenty of food with vitamin B in if you have to take antibiotics.
Found in liver, wheat germ, yeast, wholemeal bread, peas, beans.

Vitamin C does everything! – or nearly. Gums, joints, bones and teeth all need vitamin C to be healthy. Most vitamin C takers have fewer colds and flu. Research shows that people taking plenty of vitamin C have less illness.
Found in oranges, blackcurrants, grapefruit, tomatoes.

Vitamin D Your skin makes this when the sun shines on it. With the right mineral salts as well, it makes strong bones and teeth.
Found in milk, cream, butter, cheese, eggs, fish liver oil.

Vitamin E Your body uses oxygen better when it has enough of this.
Found in wheat germ.

Vitamin K helps blood clotting.
Found in leafy green vegetables.

MINERALS

Iron see page 50.

Iodine comes in sea food. You need a small amount. If you don't have enough you get a swollen, overactive thyroid gland (in your neck) called a **goitre**.

Sodium and potassium See page 77.

Calcium is needed with vitamin D for good bones and teeth.
Found in milk, yoghurt.

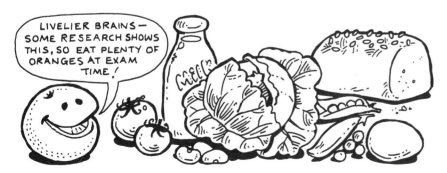

LIVELIER BRAINS—SOME RESEARCH SHOWS THIS, SO EAT PLENTY OF ORANGES AT EXAM TIME!

Babies' diets

For the first few months of life babies get all the food they need from their mothers' milk.

After that . . . raw egg, beaten into milk in a bottle, or an egg yolk stirred into hot apple puree (rather like custard!): both supply easily-digested protein and iron.

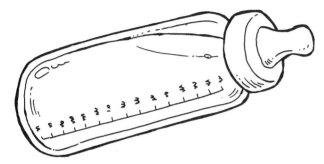

Fresh fruit juice supplies vitamin C.

Skimmed milk supplies water, and calcium salts to help bones and teeth grow healthy.

Fruit and vegetables, cooked and well mashed, will travel through babies' guts at high speed, but still supply vitamins and minerals.

Vitamins A and D may have to be added as drops but are usually already in baby milk powder.

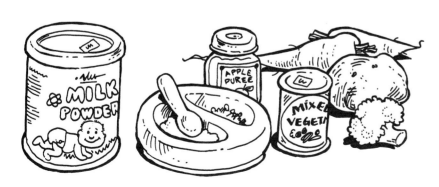

Why not sausages?

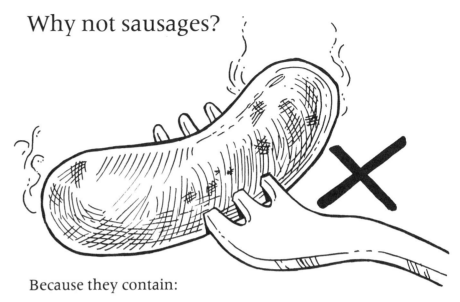

Because they contain:

(a) Fat, a big molecule needing enzymes and a fully working liver. Babies can usually digest them at one year old.

(b) Protein: more big molecules needing lots of enzymes to break them down. (Baby food manufacturers break down meat molecules by cooking.)

STARCH MOLECULE

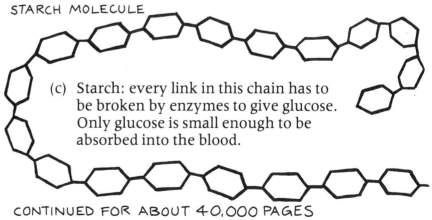

(c) Starch: every link in this chain has to be broken by enzymes to give glucose. Only glucose is small enough to be absorbed into the blood.

CONTINUED FOR ABOUT 40,000 PAGES

27

What is indigestion?

Indigestion can be a pain behind or just below the ribs, or just feeling sick.
It can be caused by:

Bacteria which can have a population explosion in
* warmed up meat pie or
* chicken not fully defrosted before cooking or
* cream cakes not kept in the refrigerator,
* and in many other foods not treated properly before you eat them.

Too much fat Liver and gall bladder can't deal with a lot of suet puddings or chips. The stomach doesn't empty and you feel full for hours after a meal.

Eating too much Don't.

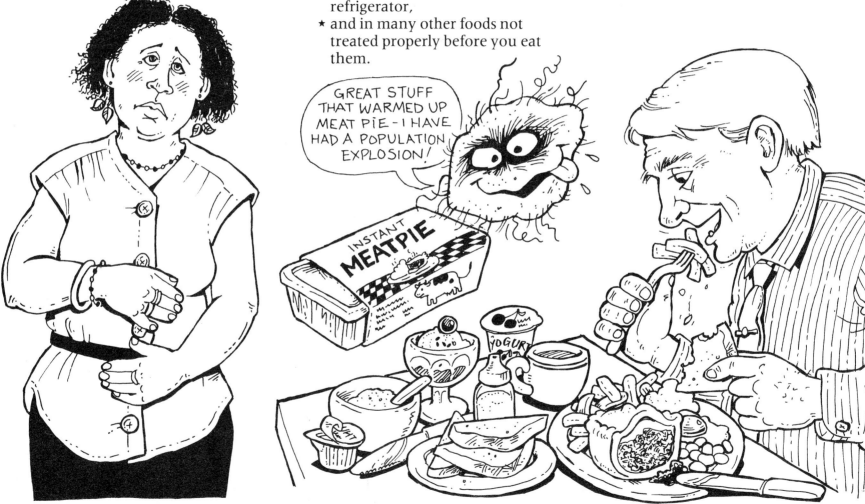

28

Acid

Your stomach makes it for:

(a) killing off some of the bacteria you eat with your food

(b) helping in the digestion of food.

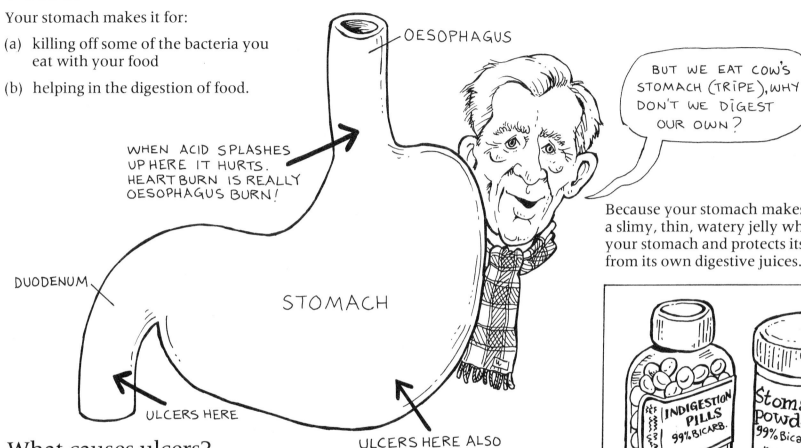

OESOPHAGUS

WHEN ACID SPLASHES UP HERE IT HURTS. HEARTBURN IS REALLY OESOPHAGUS BURN!

DUODENUM

STOMACH

ULCERS HERE

ULCERS HERE ALSO

BUT WE EAT COW'S STOMACH (TRIPE), WHY DON'T WE DIGEST OUR OWN?

Because your stomach makes mucus – a slimy, thin, watery jelly which lines your stomach and protects its walls from its own digestive juices.

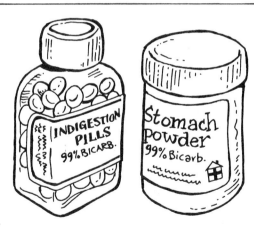

INDIGESTION PILLS 99% BICARB.

Stomach Powder 99% Bicarb.

Read the labels
Why pay twice the price for sodium bicarbonate just because it's in a fancy bottle or with some fizz?

What causes ulcers?

An ulcer is like a graze on the lining of your stomach.

1 It could be you're not making enough mucus. See your doctor.
  Or

2 You're making too much acid. This can happen if you are under strain, so stop worrying – easier said than done!

It also helps to:
drink milk and thick soups, take bicarbonate (of soda) to mop up acid, but if you take too much it wrecks your body chemistry. It is good for the occasional 'oesophagus burn', and so is milk.

Wind – what is it?

Some you swallow.

You swallow more air when:

you're nervous, or
you eat fast, or
you smoke.

MUSCLES HERE SHUT OFF THE FOOD TUBE – STOPS STOMACH ACID DAMAGING THE FOOD TUBE LINING

WIND BLOWS UP YOUR BOWELS. THE PRESSURE CAUSES PAIN.

1 The food tube muscles relax. Peppermint can help do this and so can liqueurs! That's why you have them after a meal. Things which relax these muscles are called carminatives. They make you burp.

Carminatives:
gripe water – 0 to 18 months,
peppermint – 18 months to 18 years,
Benedictine – 18 years to 80 years.

2 You lie on your left side and press the wind out of the bubble in your stomach.

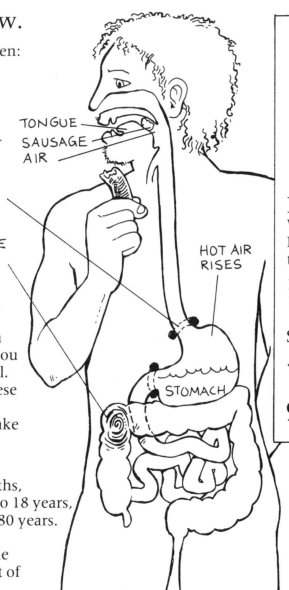

TONGUE
SAUSAGE
AIR

HOT AIR RISES

STOMACH

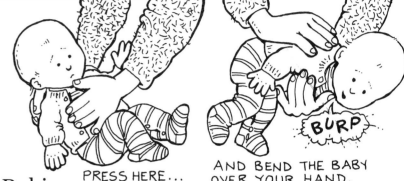

PRESS HERE...

AND BEND THE BABY OVER YOUR HAND.

BURP

Babies

Why not de-burp a baby over your shoulder?
It works in the same way but any milk that comes up with the wind goes down your back!

How do you know if a baby's got wind?
Where there's noise, there's wind!

Some people say de-burping babies doesn't matter

1 When my stomach is full of wind I can't drink any more – same with babies, so they get hungrier sooner.

2 When my intestines are full of wind it hurts. When babies feel pain they cry – so what do you think?

Sometimes, when you run, your stomach makes sloshing noises – that means there's gas in your stomach. So if you hear sloshing, de-burp.

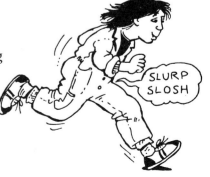

SLURP SLOSH

Wind – some you make

Yes it's microbes again, but this time your friendly local **symbiotic bacteria** (living with and helping you). They raise big families in your large intestine and give you vitamins (and wind) in return.

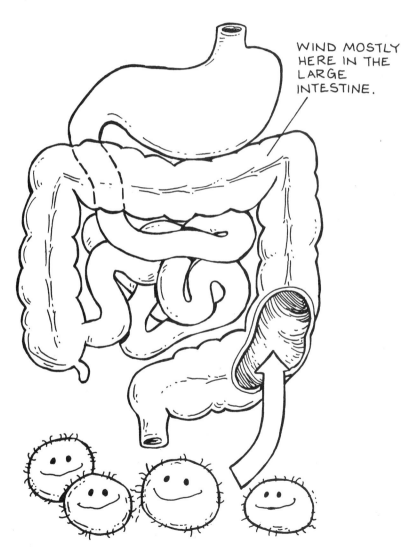

WIND MOSTLY HERE IN THE LARGE INTESTINE.

Wind is variable

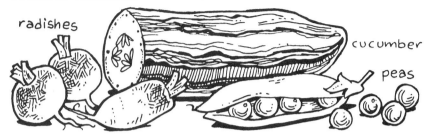

radishes
cucumber
peas

These make some people burp and some others get painful wind. But all healthy people should be able to eat a small amount without any trouble. It's all part of a well-balanced diet.

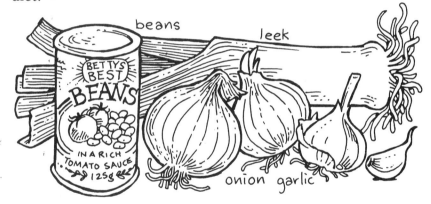

beans
leek
BETTYS BEST BEANS IN A RICH TOMATO SAUCE 125g
onion garlic

Give some people lots of wind. Why?
Maybe their bacteria don't like them, or like them too much! Everybody's different. What happens in your family?

Antibiotics kill off the friendly bacteria as well as the others – so you can have the collywobbles until the friendly ones get back again. They always do.

After operations people often get wind; is it the effect of the anaesthetic or the stirring up of the intestines?

31

Diarrhoea

Something irritates your bowel: either food poisoning bacteria, or green peppers/onions/too many prunes.

What happens in your family?

Some babies can't digest carrots, others bananas.

Your bowel muscles work overtime, pushing out the remains of the food before the walls have had time to absorb the water. (If it stayed there long enough for that the food poisoning bacteria could get into your blood.)

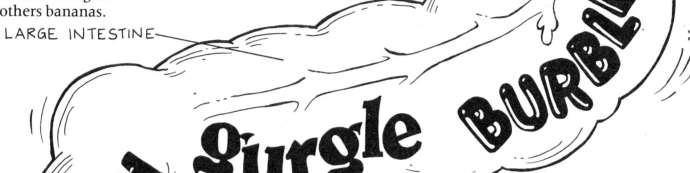

LARGE INTESTINE

WOOSH gurgle BURBLE

RECTUM

ANUS

Your bowel muscles can push so much, so hard, that they force the muscle at the end of the bowel open – then you've got the runs!

When you have diarrhoea you lose water – when you lose water you lose salt – when you lose salt you feel tired and weak.

What to do?
Well, it's better out than in!
If it goes on too long see a doctor.
If you feel tired and weak afterwards, drink some water with perhaps a dash of Ribena in it. (See page 78.)

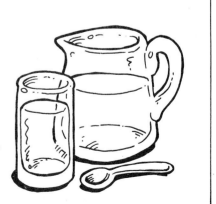

Constipation

How faeces are made

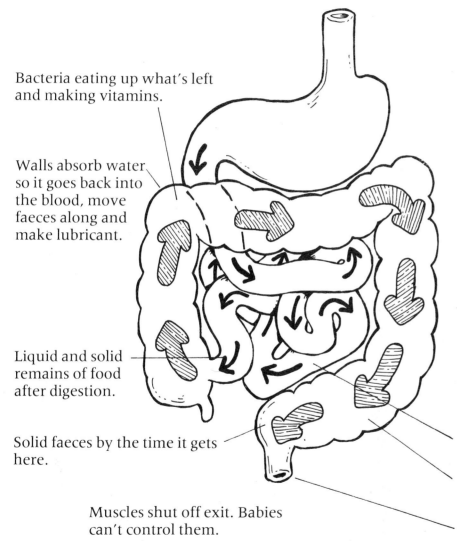

Bacteria eating up what's left and making vitamins.

Walls absorb water so it goes back into the blood, move faeces along and make lubricant.

Liquid and solid remains of food after digestion.

Solid faeces by the time it gets here.

Muscles shut off exit. Babies can't control them.

Why constipation?

Too little water
Faeces hard, muscles can't move them.
Water needed for mucous lubricant to be made.
Drink more liquid.

Too little fibre (**roughage** – undigested plant material).
Walls have nothing to grip so faeces stay put.
More water absorbed – faeces get even harder and still don't move.
Eat more cereals, vegetables and fruit – don't live on white bread and jam!

After any meal there's a mechanism at work.

Anything extra coming out of the stomach,

gives a push to what's in the intestines,

which gives a push to what's in the bowel (large intestine),

and it comes out here if you let it!

Eat plants – fibres are cheaper than laxatives.

The more plant fibres you eat, the quicker the faeces get out of your body and the healthier you are.

Straining to push out hard faeces pushes little blood vessels out of the end too! These are called **piles**. They are like small varicose veins (see page 46).

What do you have for breakfast?

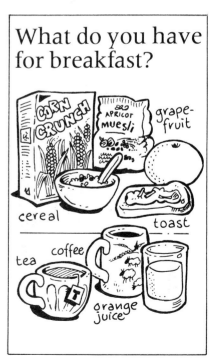

cereal

grape-fruit

toast

tea   coffee

orange juice

Check-up 2 What do you know about your teeth and digestive system?

1 Draw an idea for a poster to persuade young children to look after their teeth.
If you have some large sheets of paper you could make the poster.

2 Here are some complaints with their causes and possible cures (if any) all mixed up. Sort them out and write each one out as a complete sentence.

Example: Diarrhoea is caused by food-poisoning bacteria and is cured by drinking water with salt.

Complaint	Caused by	Helped by
Diarrhoea	making too much acid	eating more roughage
Gall stones	swallowing air with food	having an operation
Constipation	food-poisoning bacteria	eating a peppermint
Indigestion	alcohol	taking sodium bicarbonate
Cirrhosis	faeces becoming dry	stopping drinking alcohol
Stomach ulcer	crystals in gall bladder	drinking water with salt

3 Write out these sentences which are about the jobs the liver does in your body. Fill in the missing words.

(a) The gall bladder stores bile which helps dissolve ....
(b) Too much .... will give you cirrhosis of the liver.
(c) The liver stores .... as glycogen.
(d) The liver makes .... out of surplus amino acids.
(e) The liver is the largest .... in your body.

4 Copy this outline of the body and draw in the position of the parts shown.

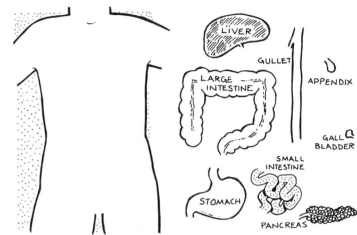

5 Copy out the table and fill in the answers.

Name of food	Vitamin in food	Vitamin's job in your body
Liver		
Carrot		
Tomato		
Egg		
Cabbage		

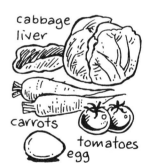

cabbage
liver
carrots
tomatoes
egg

6 Write a few sentences to explain the following.

(a) Food doesn't taste good when you have a cold.
(b) During a marathon the runners have a drink containing glucose and salt.
(c) Frozen chicken should be fully defrosted before it is cooked.
(d) Liqueurs are drunk *after* a meal.

34

Your Heart, Blood and
3 Circulation

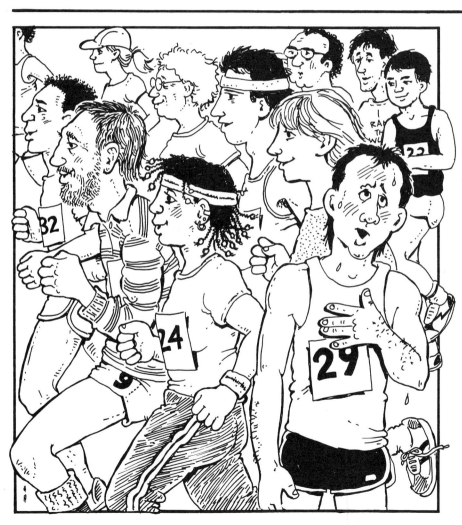

What your heart, lymph and blood do

Blood

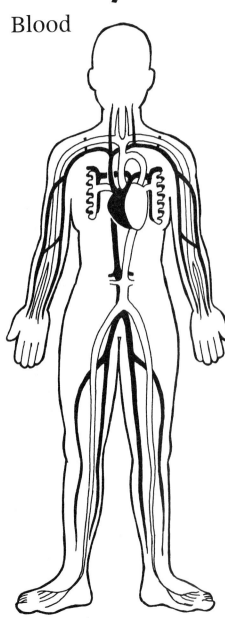

Your heart
Pumps blood around your body. Your heart must push hard enough to help get the blood back to itself. The push also squeezes **lymph** (blood without red corpuscles) out into spaces around your body cells.

Lymph
This acts as your body's drainage system. It takes proteins back from tissue spaces to blood in your veins. It takes fat from your gut to your blood system.

Lymph glands
Filter out and destroy germs and poisons and other foreign bodies from the lymph that's returning to the blood from the head, arms and legs. Lymph glands swell up when actively killing germs.

Blood
Carries around all body traffic: food, oxygen, hormones, germs, antibodies, antitoxins, water, salts, carbon dioxide, repair materials, growth materials, energy containers, cells, corpuscles, platelets.

Lymph

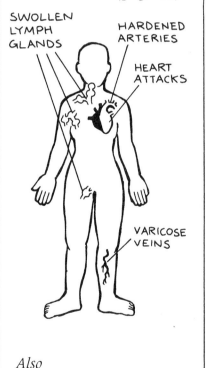

What goes wrong

Swollen lymph glands (see page 67).
Hardened arteries (maybe also blocked by cholesterol (page 44).
Heart attacks (coronary thrombosis) (page 44)
Varicose veins (page 46).

SWOLLEN LYMPH GLANDS

HARDENED ARTERIES

HEART ATTACKS

VARICOSE VEINS

Also
Anaemias (page 50)
bruises (page 52)

Your heart and how it works

Valves make sure there is only one-way traffic through your heart. If your heart is faulty and blood with carbon dioxide in it mixes with the oxygen-loaded blood, you can't walk more than a few yards.

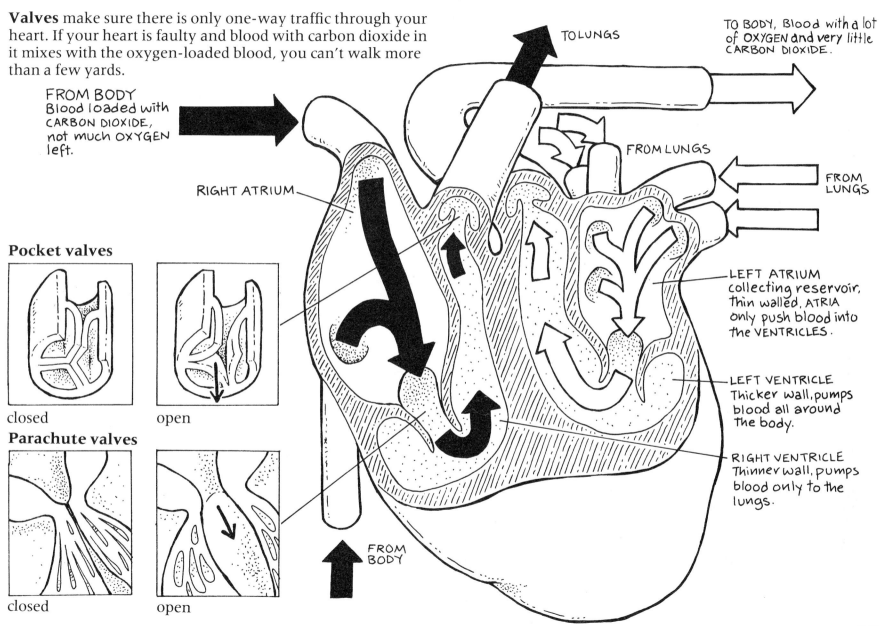

FROM BODY
Blood loaded with CARBON DIOXIDE, not much OXYGEN left.

TO LUNGS

TO BODY, Blood with a lot of OXYGEN and very little CARBON DIOXIDE.

FROM LUNGS

FROM LUNGS

RIGHT ATRIUM

LEFT ATRIUM
collecting reservoir, thin walled. ATRIA only push blood into the VENTRICLES.

LEFT VENTRICLE
Thicker wall, pumps blood all around the body.

RIGHT VENTRICLE
Thinner wall, pumps blood only to the lungs.

FROM BODY

Pocket valves

closed   open

Parachute valves

closed   open

How the blood goes round

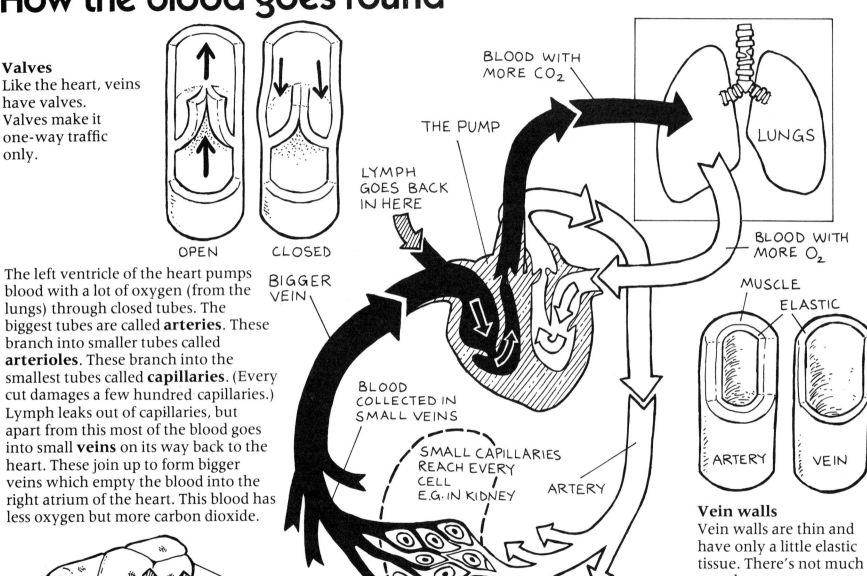

Valves
Like the heart, veins have valves. Valves make it one-way traffic only.

OPEN   CLOSED

The left ventricle of the heart pumps blood with a lot of oxygen (from the lungs) through closed tubes. The biggest tubes are called **arteries**. These branch into smaller tubes called **arterioles**. These branch into the smallest tubes called **capillaries**. (Every cut damages a few hundred capillaries.) Lymph leaks out of capillaries, but apart from this most of the blood goes into small **veins** on its way back to the heart. These join up to form bigger veins which empty the blood into the right atrium of the heart. This blood has less oxygen but more carbon dioxide.

BLOOD WITH MORE CO_2

THE PUMP

LYMPH GOES BACK IN HERE

BIGGER VEIN

LUNGS

BLOOD WITH MORE O_2

MUSCLE
ELASTIC

ARTERY   VEIN

BLOOD COLLECTED IN SMALL VEINS

SMALL CAPILLARIES REACH EVERY CELL E.G. IN KIDNEY

ARTERY

ARTERIOLE

CAPILLARY
LYMPH LEAKING OUT

Vein walls
Vein walls are thin and have only a little elastic tissue. There's not much muscle.

How does the blood get back up from your toes?

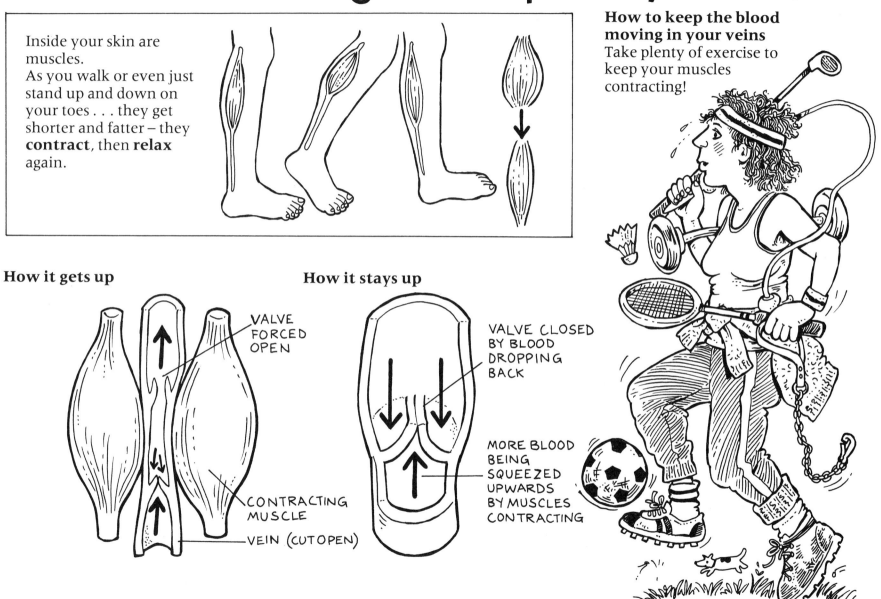

Inside your skin are muscles.
As you walk or even just stand up and down on your toes . . . they get shorter and fatter – they **contract**, then **relax** again.

How to keep the blood moving in your veins
Take plenty of exercise to keep your muscles contracting!

How it gets up

VALVE FORCED OPEN

CONTRACTING MUSCLE

VEIN (CUT OPEN)

How it stays up

VALVE CLOSED BY BLOOD DROPPING BACK

MORE BLOOD BEING SQUEEZED UPWARDS BY MUSCLES CONTRACTING

39

Why guardsmen faint

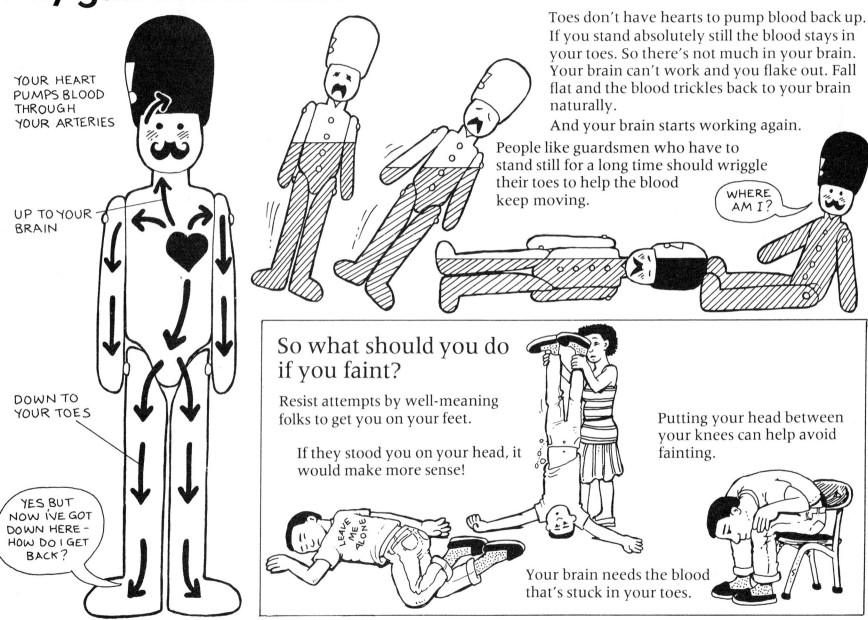

YOUR HEART PUMPS BLOOD THROUGH YOUR ARTERIES

UP TO YOUR BRAIN

DOWN TO YOUR TOES

YES BUT NOW I'VE GOT DOWN HERE — HOW DO I GET BACK?

Toes don't have hearts to pump blood back up. If you stand absolutely still the blood stays in your toes. So there's not much in your brain. Your brain can't work and you flake out. Fall flat and the blood trickles back to your brain naturally.

And your brain starts working again.

People like guardsmen who have to stand still for a long time should wriggle their toes to help the blood keep moving.

WHERE AM I?

So what should you do if you faint?

Resist attempts by well-meaning folks to get you on your feet.

If they stood you on your head, it would make more sense!

Putting your head between your knees can help avoid fainting.

LEAVE ME ALONE

Your brain needs the blood that's stuck in your toes.

40

Blue babies

Blood with plenty of oxygen in it is bright red. Oxygen is needed in your body to move muscles, to kill germs and for growth, as well as for many other things. When your blood returns to your heart from your body it has much less oxygen and a lot more carbon dioxide in it. It is a darker red, or blue-red, colour.

In blue babies the two streams of blood get mixed up. So the blood going to the body still has carbon dioxide in it and not so much oxygen. The darker red colour of this blood shows through the skin of the cheeks as a purplish blue. Blue babies can move, but not a lot, and their bodies can kill some germs, but not many, because they do not have enough oxygen going round them.

Two of the heart valves. These sometimes cause trouble in babies too. They may not close properly, so blood keeps going backwards and forwards instead of in a one-way traffic system.

One sort of hole in the heart where blood with more CO_2 in it mixes with blood with more O_2 in it. A blue baby may have this. Doctors may operate and sew up the hole.

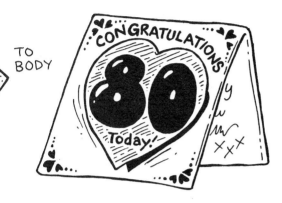

TO LUNGS

FROM BODY

FROM LUNGS

TO BODY

Darker red blood stays on one side of the heart and is pumped to the lungs where a new load of oxygen is taken on and the carbon dioxide is let out.

CONGRATULATIONS
80
Today!

Some hearts beat for 80 years without a repair man!

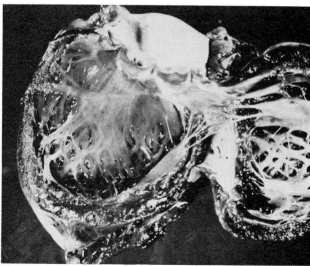

Heart cut open

What is your pulse?

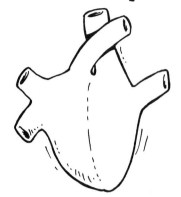

Your heart pushes blood out and your elastic artery walls stretch.

Your **pulse** is blood surging through your arteries. Your heart pushes the blood into the arteries. Their walls bulge out (as long as they're elastic). Then, while the heart is filling up again, the elastic springs back into place and the blood gets another little push on its way. Some of the energy of your heart's push is stored in the elastic walls of your arteries.
It's like pulling back the elastic of a catapult. Let go, and the energy sends the stone flying.
The push of the artery wall is what you feel as your pulse.

42

Your heart stops pushing and fills up again. The elastic wall of your artery springs back into place and gives the blood a push as it does.

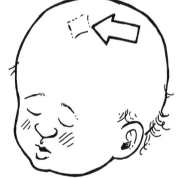

You can see a pulse on top of a baby's head, before its skull bones have joined up.

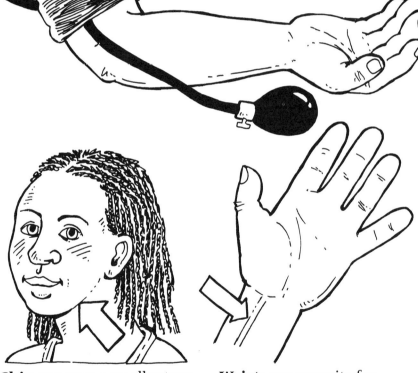

Upper arm: doctors press this artery against the bone to stop blood flow for a few seconds before they measure blood pressure. (They use a cuff, or arm band, which they blow up with a pump.)

Chin groove: a small artery crosses the bone here.

Wrist: see opposite for exactly how to find this.

You can feel a pulse when you press an artery against a bone. Try the points shown above.

Taking your own pulse

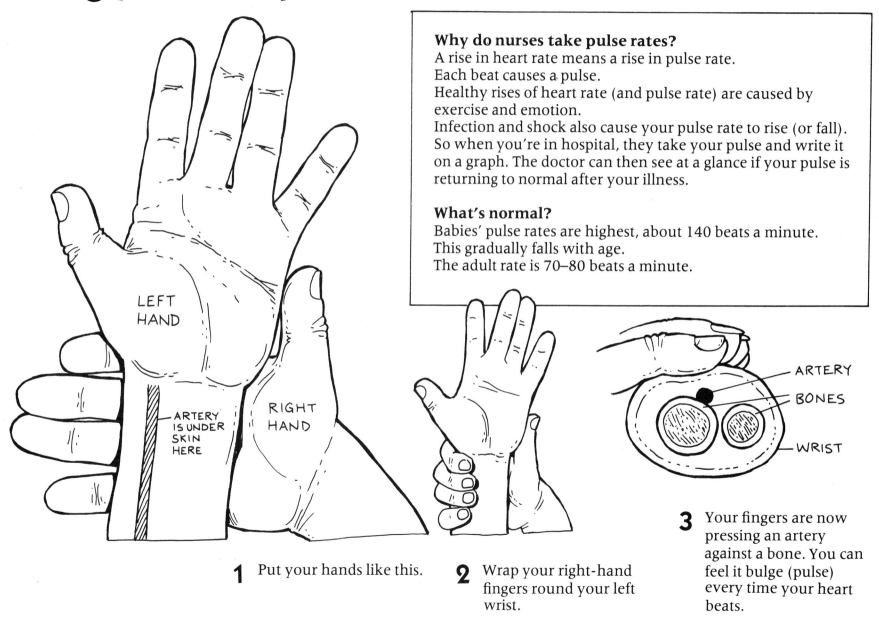

LEFT HAND

ARTERY IS UNDER SKIN HERE

RIGHT HAND

Why do nurses take pulse rates?
A rise in heart rate means a rise in pulse rate.
Each beat causes a pulse.
Healthy rises of heart rate (and pulse rate) are caused by exercise and emotion.
Infection and shock also cause your pulse rate to rise (or fall).
So when you're in hospital, they take your pulse and write it on a graph. The doctor can then see at a glance if your pulse is returning to normal after your illness.

What's normal?
Babies' pulse rates are highest, about 140 beats a minute.
This gradually falls with age.
The adult rate is 70–80 beats a minute.

ARTERY

BONES

WRIST

1 Put your hands like this.

2 Wrap your right-hand fingers round your left wrist.

3 Your fingers are now pressing an artery against a bone. You can feel it bulge (pulse) every time your heart beats.

43

Heart attacks...

The heart is a pump made of muscle which sends food and oxygen around the body in the blood. The body gets its energy from this food and oxygen. But where does the heart get its own energy from?

CORONARY ARTERY

It supplies itself with blood through this network of very thin blood vessels. These vessels are all small and narrow and are easily blocked.

The blood vessels of the heart are called **coronary blood vessels**.

Blocking one of the vessels starves the heart of food and oxygen; this means it cannot get any energy. First it goes into a kind of cramp, a pain which seems like wind but also goes along the left arm. This is a heart attack. Then, if no treatment is given, the heart may stop beating.

How do coronary blood vessels get blocked?

Coronary blood vessels are very narrow.

Smoking makes them even more narrow. So do worry and anxiety. Some people smoke because they are worried and anxious!

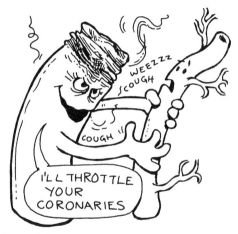

WEEZZZ
COUGH
COUGH
I'LL THROTTLE YOUR CORONARIES

Smoking
It's also expensive and gives you bronchitis.

Old age
From the ripe old age of 35 your blood vessels are less elastic so the blood can't push round any blockage in them. Alcohol hardens arteries too.

...and how to avoid them

Cholesterol

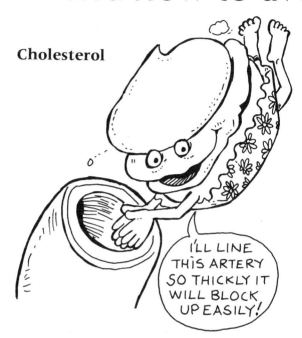

I'LL LINE THIS ARTERY SO THICKLY IT WILL BLOCK UP EASILY!

Cream cakes, pastry and sausages all contain animal fat which your body turns into **cholesterol**. This is a chemical which sticks to the inside of the arteries, narrowing them and making nice platforms on which blood clots can form very easily. Eggs contain more cholesterol than any other food – so do not eat too many.

Blood clots form easily on cholesterol linings.

Thrombosis is the long word for clot, so what's a **coronary thrombosis**?

How to stop lining your arteries with cholesterol

Cut the fat off your meat; grill fat bacon.

Use corn oil, sunflower seed oil, safflower oil (or olive oil if you can afford it!) for frying and cooking instead of lard.

Eat marge not butter, but look for these words as not all margarines are safer than butter.

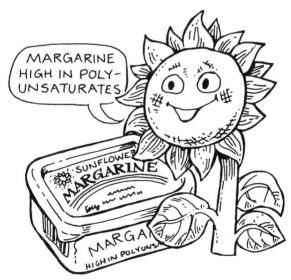

MARGARINE HIGH IN POLY-UNSATURATES

When should you begin a low cholesterol diet?

At birth – human milk is less cholesterol-producing than cow's milk – a good reason for breast feeding.

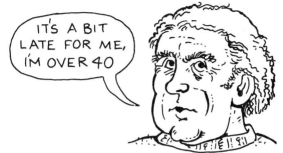

IT'S A BIT LATE FOR ME, I'M OVER 40

Better late than never

Cut down on worry, anxiety, smoking, alcohol, eggs and animal fat, and lose all that excess weight – it strains the heart.

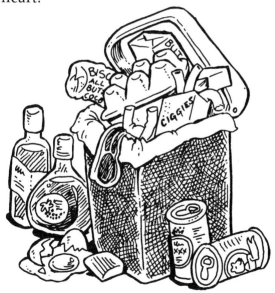

Step up exercise which keeps the blood moving so it's less likely to clot. Eat vegetable oils rather than animal fat where possible.

What are varicose veins?

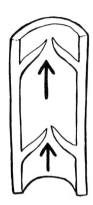

Healthy veins with

1 Strong elastic walls.

2 Valves which close, so all blood moves upwards.

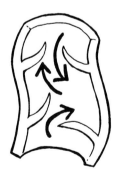

Varicose veins

1 Walls need stronger elastic!

2 Valves don't meet and blood can leak back.

What makes it happen?

Anything which keeps blood in the legs, overfills the veins and stretches the elastic until it's all broken.

Such as

Chairs like deck chairs which press right into your leg muscles and nip the veins.

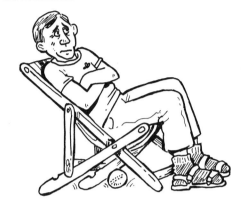

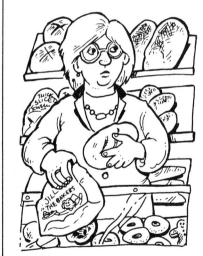

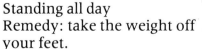

Standing all day
Remedy: take the weight off your feet.

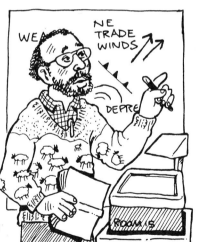

Pregnancy
The baby presses on the big veins from your legs and keeps the blood in your toes. This stretches the elastic of your veins and makes them varicose.

Standing for years
Varicose veins come on gradually if you stand up a lot at work, like teachers, or sit still, like typists.

I don't want them!

WHY?

1 They make your legs (and you) feel tired.
If the blood doesn't get back to the lungs, your leg muscles soon use all the oxygen in it. That's what feeling tired means, no oxygen for movement.
(Why do you yawn? Same reason! Your brain is not getting enough oxygen.)

2 When varicose veins are just under the skin of your legs they look like grey-blue snakes – not very pleasant!

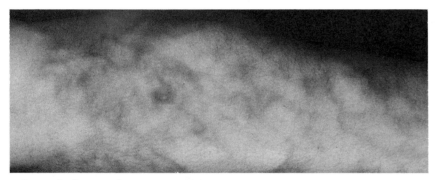

Infra-red photo of varicose veins

3 If varicose veins are cut or if an insect bites into them they can bleed badly, as there are no valves working to shut off the blood. Out it all comes from each cut end of the vein.

4 Varicose veins can be operated on, but it's not very pleasant.

5 Elastic support stockings can help sagging veins, but they are expensive, hot in summer and not very charming to look at.

SO?

Even teachers should keep moving!

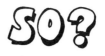

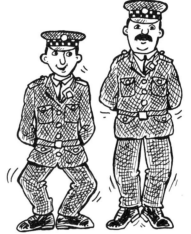

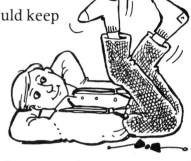

If you're going to a party and if you've been on your feet all day, 15 minutes with them **right** up, kicking about, feels great.

Always keep your legs moving. Even if you are only just going up on your toes and down again.

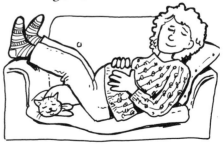

Put your feet up as often as possible. Pregnant mums should rest like this. Some people even sleep like this.

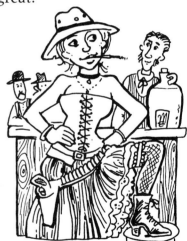

No tight girdles.

Leave garters for knights and bar girls in Western movies!

And tight boots can cause them too.

47

Blood

What is it made of?

Plasma is something like raw white of egg with water added – it has big protein molecules in it. Carbon dioxide, salts, glucose, amino acids and hormones are dissolved in it too.

Cells

White blood cells are the cleaners of your body. They eat up dead cells as well as microbes. There are about 8 thousand (8×10^3) in one small drop (1 mm³) of blood.

Red blood corpuscles carry oxygen round your body. One small drop of blood has about 5 million (5×10^6) red blood corpuscles in it.

Platelets are needed for blood clotting. One drop should have at least 250 thousand (25×10^4) of them.

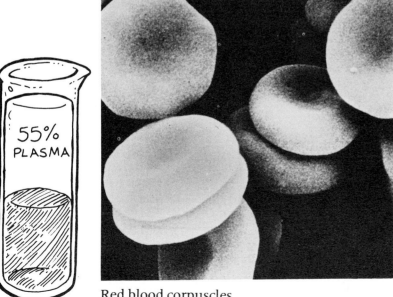

Red blood corpuscles

What does blood do?

CAPILLARY

DIGESTED FOOD FOR FUEL

OXYGEN

WATER

NERVE CELL

WATER AND IONS

PROTEIN FOR REPAIR

PROTEIN

SODIUM AND POTASSIUM IONS; NEITHER NERVES, NOR MUSCLES CAN WORK WITHOUT THESE.

BACK TO BLOOD

LYMPH VESSEL
DRAINS WATER AND PROTEIN

1 Blood carries all these things to every cell in the body through capillaries,

2 and it takes waste products away in veins.

48

Red blood corpuscles

120 days in the life of a red blood corpuscle

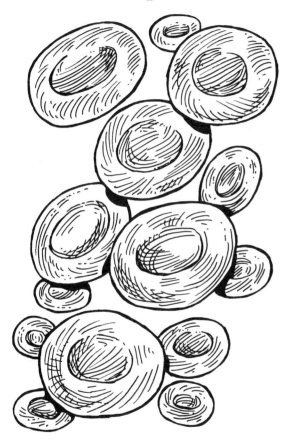

What makes them red? The oxygen-grabber, **haemoglobin**, which is red and contains iron. No iron – no oxygen-grabbing.

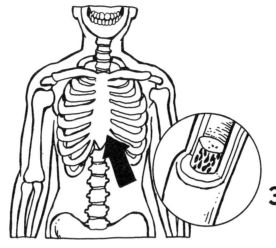

1 Born in your bone marrow. All your larger bones have marrow in them. In some illnesses doctors stick a needle in you here and take a small sample of your marrow. They look at it under a microscope to see if it's doing its job properly.

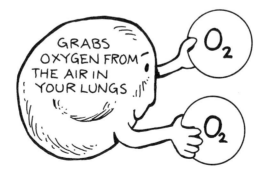

2 Goes to your lungs. Grabs oxygen from the air in your lungs.

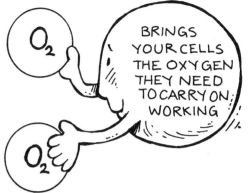

3 Pumped by your heart to your muscles, skin, bone, teeth, stomach, bladder, eyes, ears, and everywhere. Brings your cells the oxygen they need to carry on working.

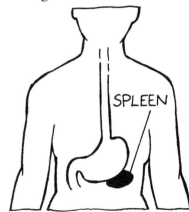

4 Has 120 days (more or less) hard labour going round and round. Flakes out in the spleen – the graveyard of the red corpuscles – and is broken down to help make new red corpuscles.

Anaemia

This is when you don't have enough red blood corpuscles. It can be caused by all sorts of things. The most common kind happens when girls and women lose blood regularly during menstruation and do not eat enough iron-containing foods to replace the red blood corpuscles.

 Pull down your lower eyelid. If it's red inside – O.K.

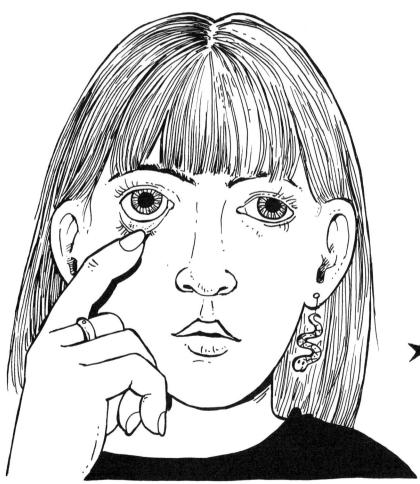

 If it's pink – you could eat more

Curry
Black treacle
Oatmeal
Soya flour
Red meat
Liver
Kidneys
Corned beef
or even, cockles, mussels, winkles
Black pudding – slice and grill it!

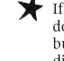
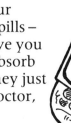

 If it's pale, almost white, see your doctor, who may give you iron pills – but don't be surprised if they give you diarrhoea! Some people don't absorb the iron pills into their blood; they just go straight through. Tell your doctor, who'll change the treatment.

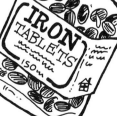

Antibodies

Antibodies are made by white blood cells.

They wrap up Fred the germ and his relations and put them out of action.

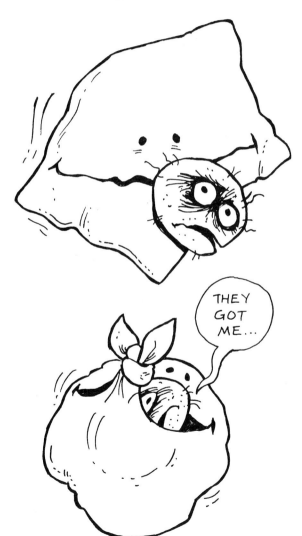

THEY GOT ME...

Healthy people make most of their own antibodies but even healthy people need help.

Dead germs – to make their bodies 'think' they need to make antibodies, so they do. Then the antibodies are ready if some real live germs get in later.

Someone else's antibodies can be given when it is too late to wait for your own body to make antibodies. (Used against tetanus.)

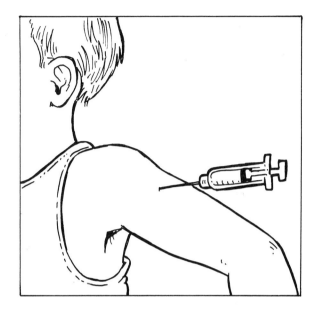

Antigen – something which stirs up the body to make an antibody; in this case the antigen is the flu virus.

Injections of dead, clean, flu viruses grown in hens' eggs help stop people catching flu.

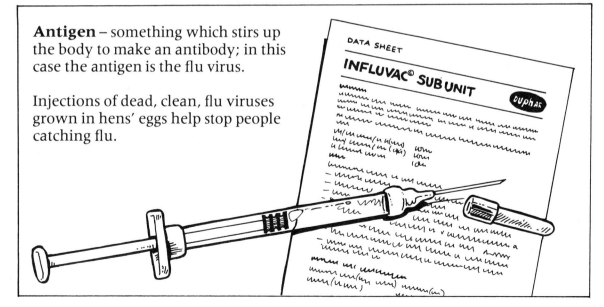

DATA SHEET

INFLUVAC© SUB UNIT

DUPHAR

Cuts and bruises

Cuts

Red blood corpuscles rarely leave blood vessels except when the skin is cut.

This is Fred. He is a **germ**, and there are a lot of him around.
If Fred gets in, he starts to raise a large family. But white blood cells eat up as many Freds as they can. Some white cells die doing this.

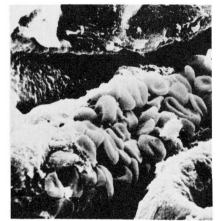

Red blood corpuscles densely packed into blood capillary

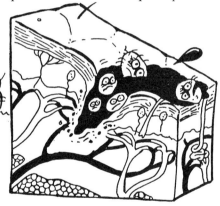

What to do

If it's a small cut let it bleed – this washes away the Freds. Don't grind them in with a dirty hankie. When the blood clots, wash away dried blood from around the cut and cover with a plaster.

Bruises

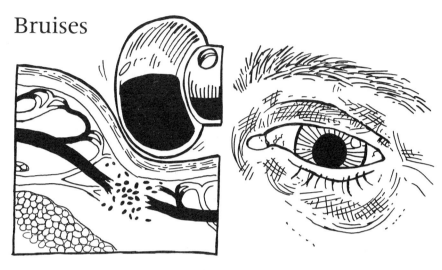

Red blood corpuscles can leave blood vessels when the vessels are broken without the skin being cut.
This is a bruise:
First it's red as the red cells flow out of the broken vessels, then the red cells start to die and the bruise turns purple, then yellow.
The white blood cells are doing the work. They eat up dead red corpuscles and make the purple and yellow colours.
Don't waste steak on a black eye! Eat it – it will help to replace those dead red blood corpuscles.

What to do with a bruise

1 While it's red apply something cold. This makes the blood vessels contract, so less blood leaks out.

2 While it's purple or green give it heat. Blood vessels have healed up by now and heat makes the tropical sunset go quicker!

Clotting

When you cut yourself

1 A clotting chemical is released from your damaged cells and your platelets, which break open.

2 This chemical acts with other chemicals to turn one of the proteins in your plasma into threads (like hot fat acts on egg-white).

3 These threads close the cut, catching red blood corpuscles, which give the clot its colour, and white cells too.

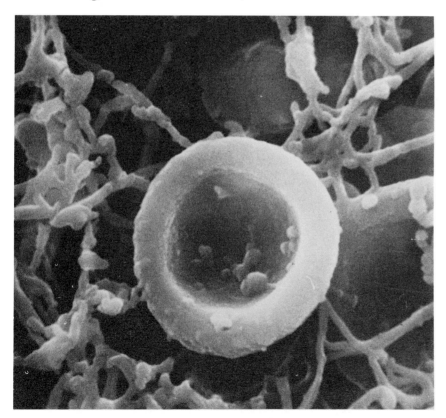

Network of fibrin traps red blood corpuscles

Unfortunately, blood clots can form inside blood vessels, even when they are not cut or bruised.

A thrombosis is a clot (see page 45).

Sticky platelets gather inside the blood vessel. The more fat there is in the blood, the easier it is for the platelets to stick together. People who eat lots of cream, sausages, fat meat and pastry are likely to get more blood clots inside their blood vessels. So are people who are overweight.

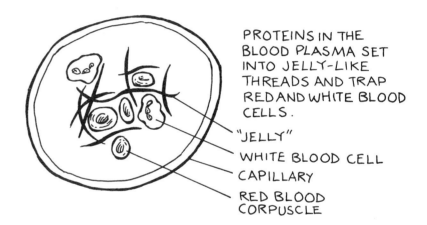

PROTEINS IN THE BLOOD PLASMA SET INTO JELLY-LIKE THREADS AND TRAP RED AND WHITE BLOOD CELLS.

"JELLY"

WHITE BLOOD CELL

CAPILLARY

RED BLOOD CORPUSCLE

When a clot inside a blood vessel breaks off and travels around your blood vessels, it soon reaches one which it can block. Maybe in your brain, so you have a stroke; maybe in your coronary artery so your heart is starved of oxygen and you have a heart attack.

After surgery or having a baby
The nurses get you out of bed quickly – this is not because they are unkind or heartless. You may not feel like walking or even sitting, but any exercise helps to get your circulation going and you are less likely to get a clot, thrombosis or embolism, whatever you like to call it.

53

Blood groups and transfusions

Do you know your blood group?

Probably not unless you have had a transfusion or are a blood donor and have a card like this.

You can be a donor when you are 18 so long as you haven't had hepatitis or malaria, or don't have AIDs!

What are blood groups?

Different substances on your red corpuscles and in your plasma give you your blood group.

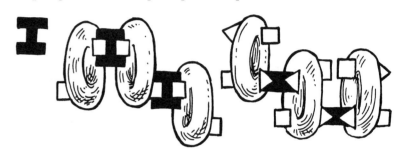

NATIONAL BLOOD TRANSFUSION SERVICE

Blood group A   RH. POSITIVE

CHECK GROUP BEFORE TRANSFUSION

Issued by NORTH LONDON BLOOD TRANSFUSION CENTRE
DEANSBROOK ROAD
EDGWARE MIDDLESEX HA8 9BD
Tel 01·952 5511
DONOR'S SIGNATURE   N.B.T.S.107(A)P   DATE

Plasma has substances called **antibodies** in it; these may be anti-A or anti-B. Antibodies make corpuscles of the right kind clump together or they may destroy them.

Anti-A will clump corpuscles which have A (blood groups A and AB).

Anti-B will clump corpuscles which have B (groups B and AB) in the same way.

You do not normally have an antibody that clumps your own red corpuscles in your blood.

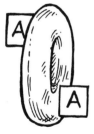

If you are blood group A, you have a chemical substance A on your red corpuscles.

If both substances are present you are group AB.

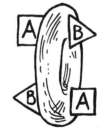

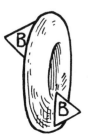

If blood group B, you have chemical substance B.

Neither – group O!

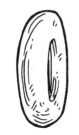

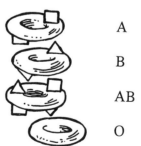

Your blood group	**Antibody in your plasma will be**
A	Anti-B
B	Anti-A
AB	Neither
O	Both

Does it matter which blood group you are?

Most of the time it doesn't but if you lose a lot of blood during an operation or in an accident, it is important that you are not given blood containing cells which your antibodies will clump. Can you see why blood group O is called the **universal donor**?

The Rhesus factor

Six out of seven people have a substance called the **Rhesus factor** in their blood; they are Rhesus positive (Rh+). If you don't have it you are Rhesus negative.

Usually people do not have an anti-Rh antibody in their blood but if Rh+ blood is given to a Rh− person in a transfusion:

No harm is done the first time but an anti-Rh antibody is formed which stays in the blood. If Rh+ blood is given a second time, the person becomes very ill.

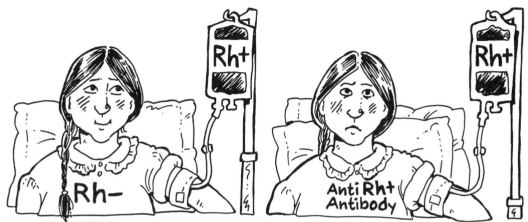

Rhesus babies

These babies are born with jaundice and anaemia. This can happen when Mum is Rh− and Dad is Rh+.
Rh− babies will be all right, so will the first Rh+ one, but its blood mixes with the mother's blood at birth. Mum makes anti-Rh antibodies to this blood. If the second baby is Rh+, it is a Rhesus baby because Mum's anti-Rh antibodies get into its blood before birth.
Its blood can be replaced with fresh blood.
Mum can also be treated now to stop it happening.

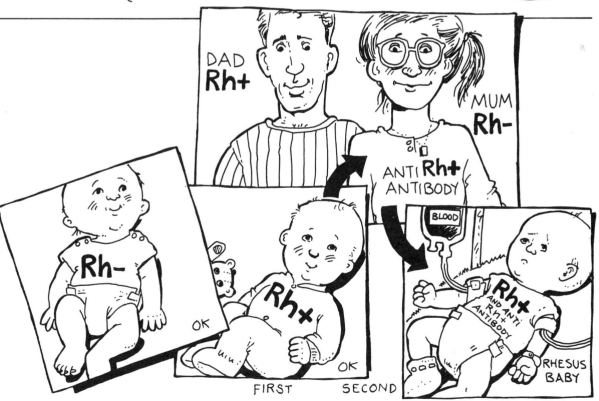

Lymph

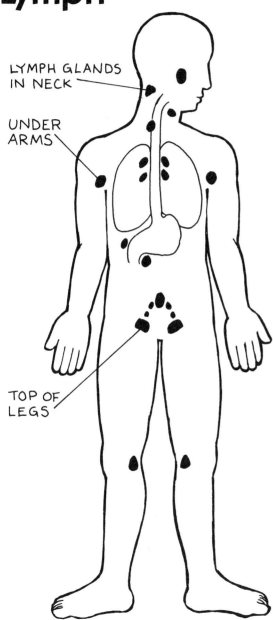

LYMPH GLANDS IN NECK

UNDER ARMS

TOP OF LEGS

Lymph is pushed out from the blood in the smallest blood vessels by pressure from the heart beating.

Which glands sometimes swell when you have a cold?
When you stand on a piece of glass?
When you cut your finger?

Lymph glands are checkpoints

They filter blood coming back from your arms, legs and head to your heart. So if you have a septic finger you don't get a septic heart, because white blood cells sit in the lymph glands waiting to eat up germs.

Glands swell when they are working hard.

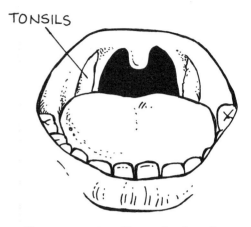

TONSILS

Tonsils are a pair of lymph glands checking the blood from your nose and throat. If there are too many germs for them to cope with you may get septic tonsils (full of dead white blood cells) and these have to be removed.

The Black Death in the 14th Century made lymph glands swell – one of the signs by which people knew they had it – but by then it was too late to do anything about it.

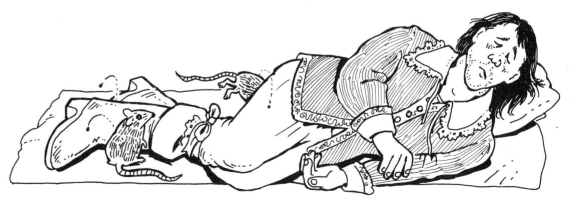

What goes wrong with it?

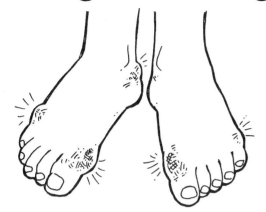

Blisters

Your new summer sandals rub against your toe.
It becomes red. Blood vessels in the area are very full and leak a lot of lymph into the pressure area, making a blister.

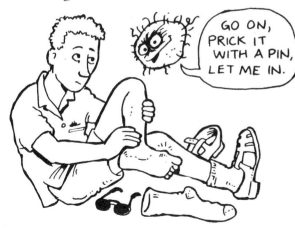

GO ON, PRICK IT WITH A PIN, LET ME IN.

Don't. Cover with a plaster and leave it alone. (Throw away those sandals.)

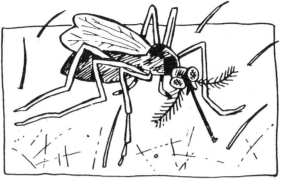

Insect bites

Insect saliva damages blood vessels and helps them leak lymph. Lymph leaks out and makes a swelling.

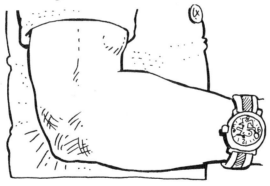

Waterlogging

Water on the knee, swollen ankles, tennis elbow.
Either the blood is not getting back to the heart properly, so more lymph leaks out of it, or there are other reasons. In any case see your doctor.

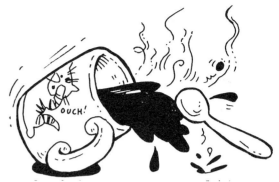

Scalds and burns

Blisters may form here too. Cold water will cool them. In bad cases see a doctor. Positively no pin pricking. Unless you want Fred to have a population explosion.

Leukaemia

If white blood cells grow very fast they take the place of red corpuscles, the oxygen-grabbers. People with **leukaemia** (cancer of white blood cells) die of oxygen-lack – their blood contains too many white cells. But white cells live in lymph glands, which can also become cancerous. Leukaemia research is helping more people live longer; soon there may be a cure for all the different kinds of cancer.
Cancer is when any body cell multiplies very fast, out of control, and makes a tumour. (See page 150.)

Check-up 3 What do you know about your heart, blood and circulation?

1 Match the correct description with the name and write out the full sentence.

Name	Description
Cholesterol	is when you do not have enough red blood cells.
Plasma	is a chemical that can cause heart attacks.
Anaemia	can put germs out of action.
Platelets	is cancer of the white blood cells.
Antibodies	is the name of a type of chamber in the heart.
Leukaemia	is the part of the blood with many things dissolved in it.
Ventricle	help the blood to clot.

2 Which of these do you think is good for you and which is bad for you? **Give your reasons why**.

Good	Bad	Reason

(a) Eating three cream cakes a day.
(b) Taking regular exercise.
(c) Smoking cigarettes.
(d) Eating foods that contain iron.
(e) Drinking lots of beer.
(f) Trying to keep your legs moving.
(g) Eating margarine that is 'high in polyunsaturates'.
(h) Not worrying.

3 Which of these statements are true and which are false?

- The heart is mostly made of muscle.
- Veins have valves in them.
- Arteries are the smallest blood vessels.
- Veins have thick muscular walls.
- Your pulse is blood surging through your arteries.
- Capillaries can carry blood containing oxygen.
- The heart has four chambers.
- Bright red blood has lots of oxygen in it.
- An arteriole is a big artery.
- The left ventricle has thin muscular walls.

4 Do you know the differences between arterial blood, venous blood and lymph?

(a) Which has few, if any, red blood corpuscles?
(b) Which has most white blood cells?
(c) Which carries most large molecules?
(d) Which has most oxygen?
(e) Which has most carbon dioxide?
(f) Which is bright red?
(g) Which is dull red?
(h) Which is colourless?

5 Write out these sentences and fill in the gaps, using the words from the box.

neck	proteins	poisons	fat	working
arms	glands	swollen	legs	

Lymph is a fluid that comes from the blood. It carries .... from spaces around the tissues back into your veins and it takes .... from your digestive system to your blood system. Small swellings called lymph .... act as a filter system. They kill germs, destroy .... and remove any foreign bodies in the lymph before it goes back into the blood. Lymph glands are found in the .... , under the .... and at the top of the .... They swell up when they are .... hard and this is why you have '.......... glands' when you are ill.

6 What causes each of these problems? Make a table like this one:

Problem	What causes the problem?

Thrombosis   Hardened arteries   Bruise
Varicose veins   Clogged coronary artery   Swollen glands

58

Your Lungs and Breathing System

4

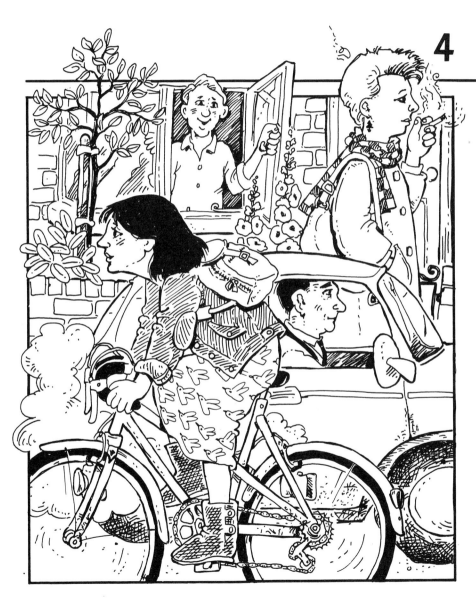

How do you get oxygen?

You need oxygen to release energy from the food you eat.

Oxygen from the air

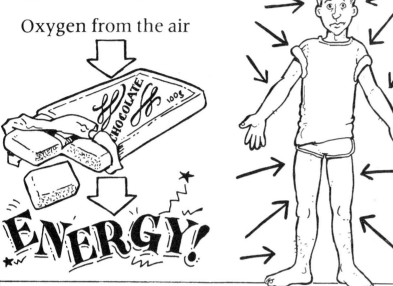

ENERGY!

Your lungs look spongy because of the millions of air sacs at the ends of the branching tubes (bronchioles).

If laid out flat, one of your lungs would cover the area of a tennis court!

The entrance to your lungs is through your nose and throat (pharynx).

Part of your breathing system

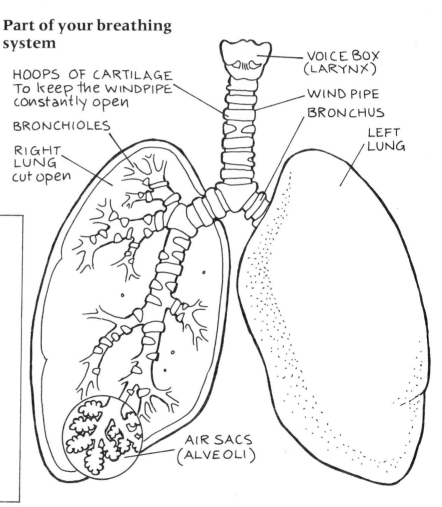

VOICE BOX (LARYNX)

HOOPS OF CARTILAGE To keep the WINDPIPE constantly open

WIND PIPE

BRONCHUS

BRONCHIOLES

LEFT LUNG

RIGHT LUNG cut open

AIR SACS (ALVEOLI)

Your surface area compared with the surface area of the beginning of your breathing system.

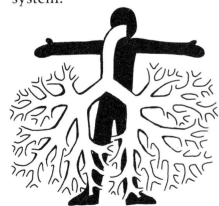

Can you get enough oxygen through your skin?

You have billions of cells inside your body which need oxygen, so the answer is no. Instead you have a huge internal surface to take in oxygen.

Most of this enormous surface is formed by your lungs.

Problems of the breathing system

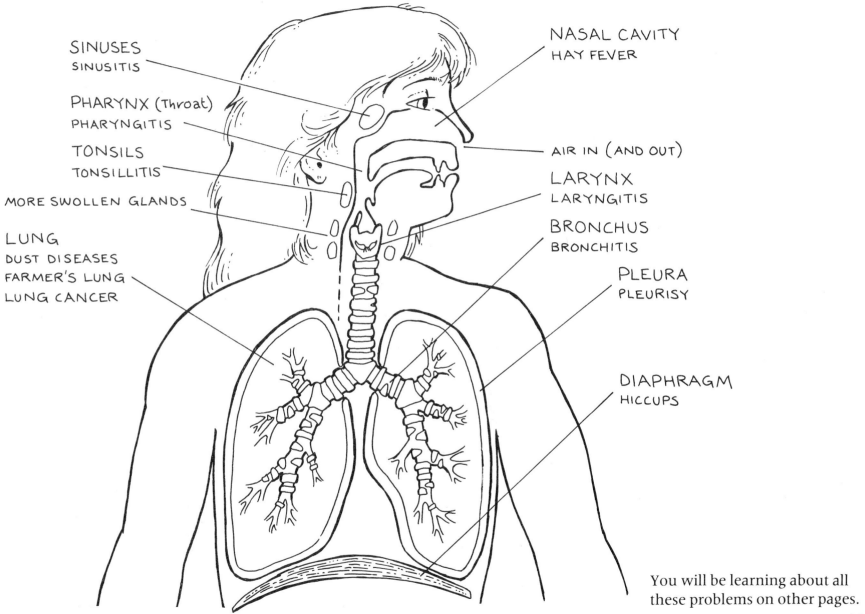

SINUSES
SINUSITIS

PHARYNX (Throat)
PHARYNGITIS

TONSILS
TONSILLITIS

MORE SWOLLEN GLANDS

LUNG
DUST DISEASES
FARMER'S LUNG
LUNG CANCER

NASAL CAVITY
HAY FEVER

AIR IN (AND OUT)

LARYNX
LARYNGITIS

BRONCHUS
BRONCHITIS

PLEURA
PLEURISY

DIAPHRAGM
HICCUPS

You will be learning about all
these problems on other pages.

61

Your own air-conditioning system

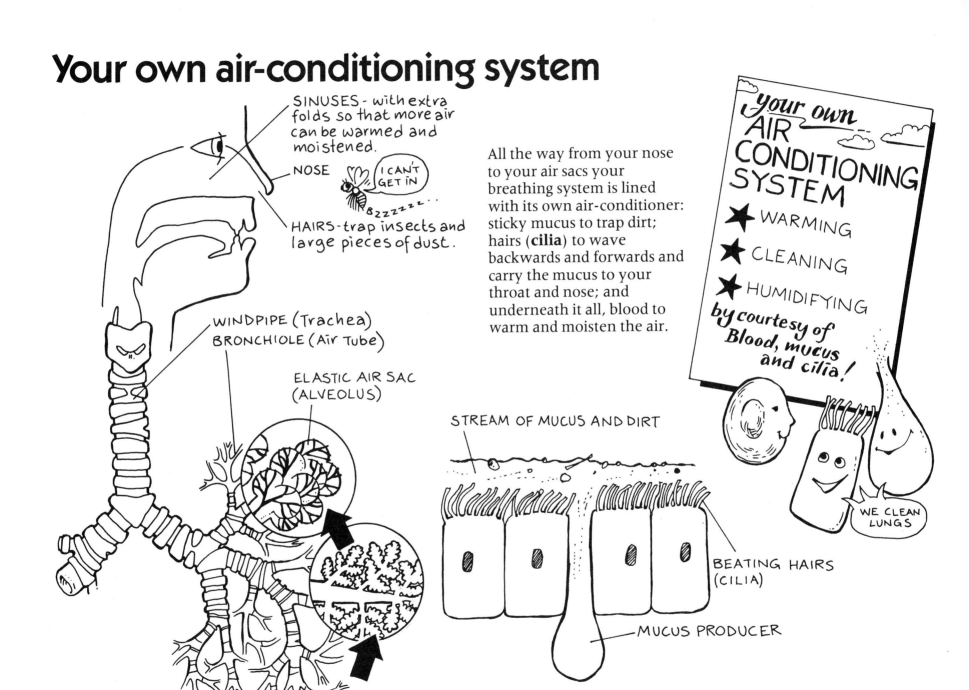

SINUSES - with extra folds so that more air can be warmed and moistened.

NOSE

I CAN'T GET IN

Bzzzzzz...

HAIRS - trap insects and large pieces of dust.

All the way from your nose to your air sacs your breathing system is lined with its own air-conditioner: sticky mucus to trap dirt; hairs (**cilia**) to wave backwards and forwards and carry the mucus to your throat and nose; and underneath it all, blood to warm and moisten the air.

WINDPIPE (Trachea)
BRONCHIOLE (Air Tube)

ELASTIC AIR SAC (ALVEOLUS)

STREAM OF MUCUS AND DIRT

BEATING HAIRS (CILIA)

MUCUS PRODUCER

your own AIR CONDITIONING SYSTEM
★ WARMING
★ CLEANING
★ HUMIDIFYING
by courtesy of Blood, mucus and cilia!

WE CLEAN LUNGS

The kiss of life

Before starting make sure there's no water in the lungs, there's nothing blocking the throat.

1 Lie the patient on his/her back.

2 Bend the head back to open the air passages.

3 Pinch the nose closed so no air escapes here.

4 Blow through the mouth; feel the ribs rise with the other hand.

5 Stop blowing and let the air come out; help this if necessary by pressing on the chest.

6 Keep repeating steps 3 and 4 every 4–6 seconds.

When you blow in, the air sacs inflate and the chest wall rises.
When you stop blowing the air sacs deflate and the chest wall falls (by itself usually) and pushes air out.

Keep the patient warm.

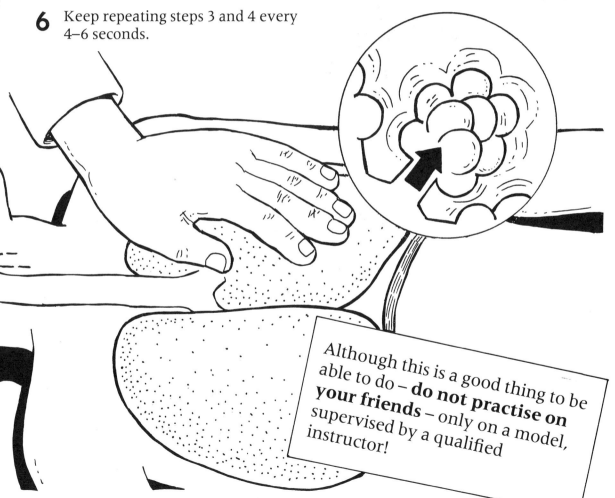

Although this is a good thing to be able to do – **do not practise on your friends** – only on a model, supervised by a qualified instructor!

Hiccups!

Jack O'Leary of Los Angeles 'hicked' 160 000 000 times from 13 June 1948 to 1 June 1956 with a week off in 1951. He lost over 4 stone. A prayer to St Jude apparently cured him.

(Guinness Book of Records)

What makes you hiccup? – hiccough?

☆ Too-hot drinks?

☆ Peppery food?

☆ Laughing?

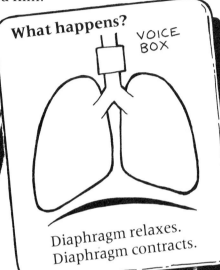

What happens?

VOICE BOX

Diaphragm relaxes.
Diaphragm contracts.

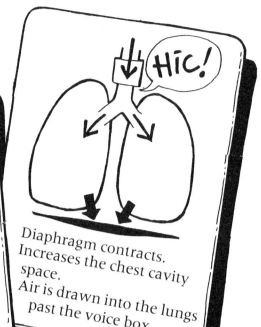

HIC!

Diaphragm contracts.
Increases the chest cavity space.
Air is drawn into the lungs past the voice box.

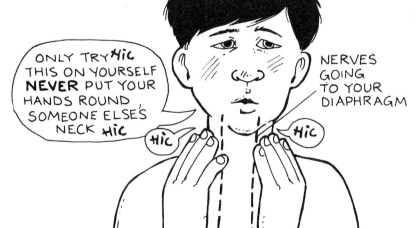

ONLY TRY HIC THIS ON YOURSELF **NEVER** PUT YOUR HANDS ROUND SOMEONE ELSE'S NECK HIC

HIC

HIC

NERVES GOING TO YOUR DIAPHRAGM

How to stop

1 Take a deep breath and hold it.

2 Press your fingers hard into your neck where those nerves are.

3 Let your breath out when you have to. Has it stopped?

4 No? Do it again. You were too giggly the first time.

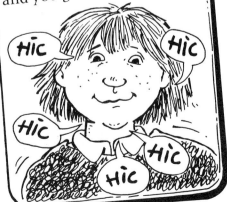

And the diaphragm goes on with short sharp contractions and you go on hiccupping!

HIC HIC HIC HIC HIC

Model hiccups

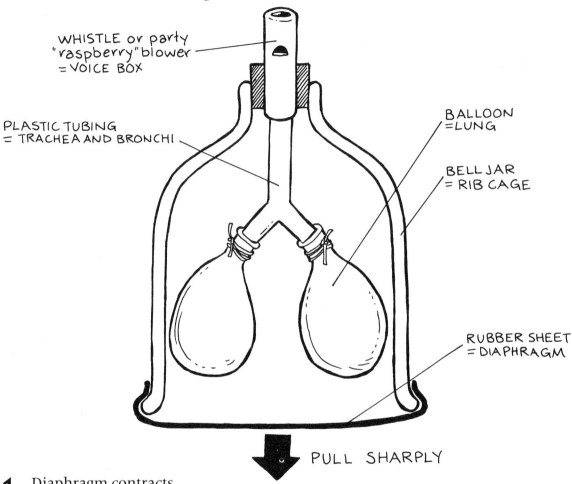

WHISTLE or party "raspberry" blower = VOICE BOX

PLASTIC TUBING = TRACHEA AND BRONCHI

BALLOON = LUNG

BELL JAR = RIB CAGE

RUBBER SHEET = DIAPHRAGM

PULL SHARPLY

1 Diaphragm contracts.

2 Chest cavity space increases.

3 Lungs have quick intake of air.

4 Voice box hiccups!

Now make a list of all the ways in which the model is different from the real thing.

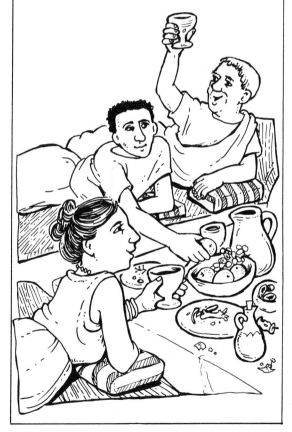

Bit of history
The nerve you press to make yourself stop hiccupping is the same one that the Romans and the City of London Aldermen used to tickle gently to make themselves sick. Why? So that they could eat more at their banquets! No kidding.

Lungs and lymph

Your lungs inside your chest cavity fill with air then empty all day and all night – for 75 years or even more!

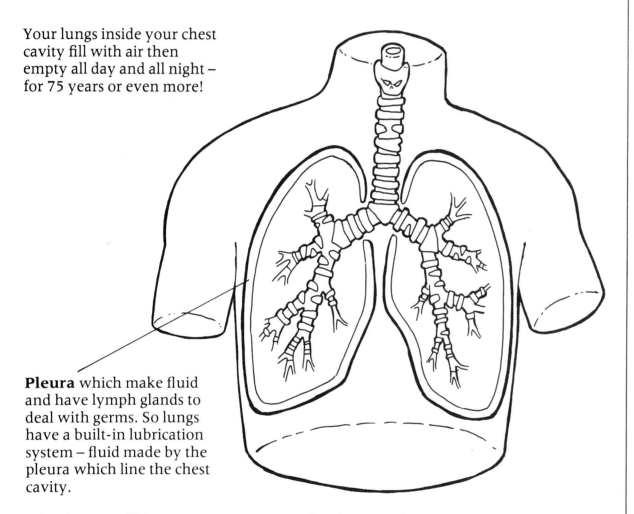

Pleura which make fluid and have lymph glands to deal with germs. So lungs have a built-in lubrication system – fluid made by the pleura which line the chest cavity.

What happens if the germs win?

You get pleurisy. Your lungs creak and scratch against your ribs because your pleura are too busy fighting germs to make fluid.

Lungs and smoking

Some people smoke all their lives and never get lung cancer.

All smokers get the wheezes and the '-itises'.

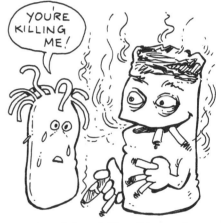

YOU'RE KILLING ME!

True. Smoking kills cilia so they can't waft the muck and mucus out. It stays there, stuck in the air tubes, and wheezes every time the air goes in and out.

Ever heard a smoker clearing his throat first thing in the morning? That muck and mucus has been trying to get out all night!

Bronchitis is more common and just as unpleasant as lung cancer.

Kill your cilia and you'll get it!

'Itises'

When germs get into a part of your body and blood rushes to your body's defence.

Sinusitis

What to do

1 Keep warm, breathe warm air.

2 Drink warm drinks.

What do sinuses do?
They

1 warm up,

2 clean, and

3 moisten the air you take in.

So your lungs only get ready-warmed, slightly damp air with most of the dirt and germs taken out. When the air gets into your lungs the only body defences left to fight germs are your white cells and antibodies in your blood – and also your lymph glands in your pleura (the lining of your chest).

Bronchitis
What to do

1 Stay in bed and keep warm.

2 Call a doctor.

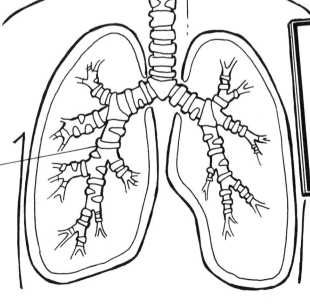

Sore throat – pharyngitis and tonsillitis

Red tonsils, due to blood rushing to your defence.
Tonsils are lymph glands. Sometimes they swell up from working so hard trying to kill germs. Sometimes the germs win and your tonsils have to be taken out.
All the other '-itises' look red too and maybe swollen, but you can't always see them.

Laryngitis

What to do

1 Stop talking.

2 Drink warm drinks.

Smokers get more '-itises' than anyone else (except appendicitis!)

Smoking lowers your body defences against germs – makes your air-conditioning cilia work overtime, eventually paralyses them and affects the mucus flow.

What's **inflammation**? Redness.
What's it due to? Blood vessels opening up and filling with blood.
Why? To bring your white cells and antibodies to fight the germs.

Why do people wear masks?

When the cleaning mechanism of the lungs isn't enough.

Against germs

Doctors and nurses wear them to stop germs from their noses and mouths getting on to people having operations or on to newborn babies.

Air pollution

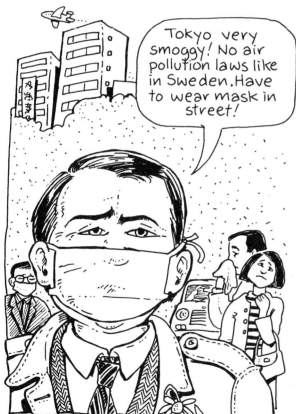

Tokyo very smoggy! No air pollution laws like in Sweden. Have to wear mask in street!

Industry

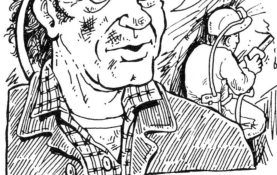

Well no, I don't wear a mask - but maybe I should, X-rays show my lungs are full of coal dust.

Silica dust in South Wales coal really damages lungs – tears them to bits. Miners do wear masks there.

Country dust

Jarge, he just can't go out of the house at hay harvest time, never mind wear a mask.

Dust from hay, wheat and fungus can all damage the lung-cleaning mechanism of people working on farms – gives a disease called farmer's lung, which is like bronchitis but worse.

Getting things out of your lungs

Sneezing

Air is forced out through your nose and sometimes takes what's irritating you with it. (But some people sneeze when they see the sun – do you?)

Water comes out of your lungs at all these points. Nose, windpipe and air tubes all make mucus; this takes a lot of water. When you've got a cold, the germs irritate the mucus-making glands and the mucus is even more watery.

The air coming from the air sacs is warmer as well as wetter.

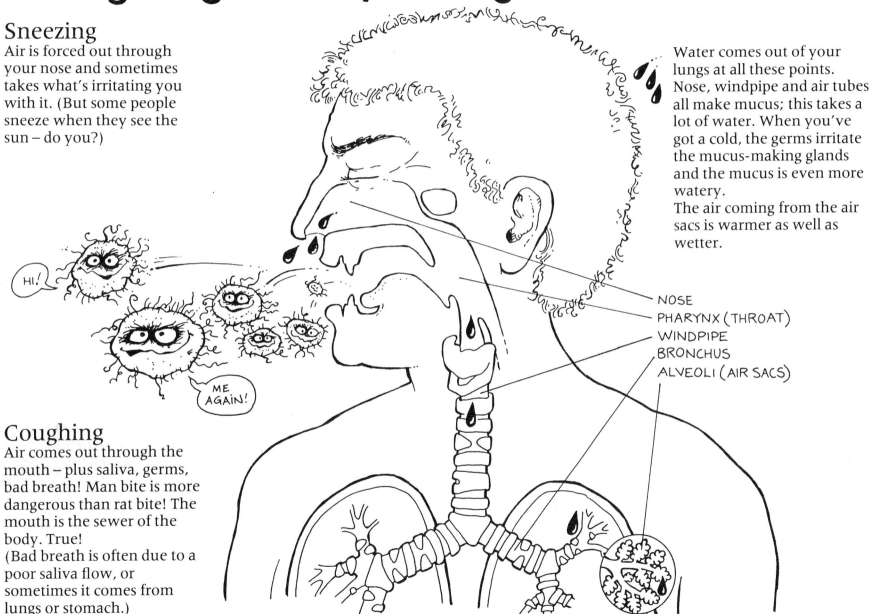

HI!

ME AGAIN!

NOSE
PHARYNX (THROAT)
WINDPIPE
BRONCHUS
ALVEOLI (AIR SACS)

Coughing

Air comes out through the mouth – plus saliva, germs, bad breath! Man bite is more dangerous than rat bite! The mouth is the sewer of the body. True!
(Bad breath is often due to a poor saliva flow, or sometimes it comes from lungs or stomach.)

Carbon dioxide and carbon monoxide

Chest cavity gets bigger – air goes in.

More oxygen in air going in – grabbed by haemoglobin in red blood corpuscles.

Chest cavity gets smaller – air goes out.

More carbon dioxide in air going out – released from blood plasma which has collected it from all the cells in your body.

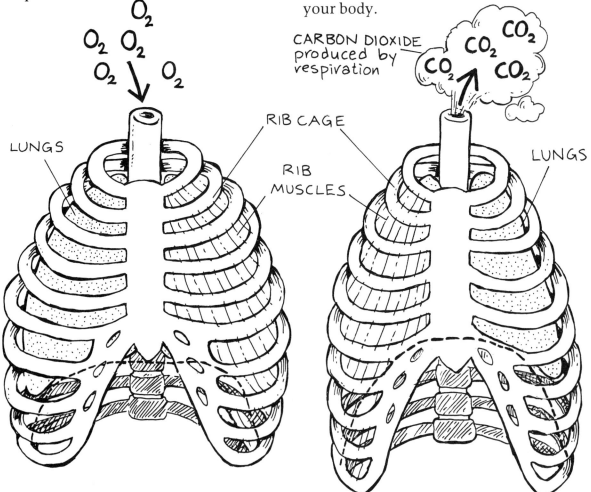

O_2 O_2 O_2 O_2 O_2

LUNGS

RIB CAGE

RIB MUSCLES

CARBON DIOXIDE produced by respiration

CO_2 CO_2 CO_2 CO_2 CO_2

LUNGS

DIAPHRAGM

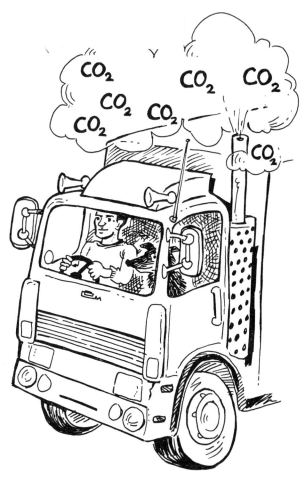

CO_2 CO_2 CO_2 CO_2 CO_2 CO_2 CO_2

CO, carbon **mon**oxide, produced by petrol and diesel engines.
Red blood corpuscles will grab it instead of oxygen, so never run an engine in a closed garage. You could replace all the oxygen in your red blood corpuscles with carbon monoxide and die.

Lung defences

Defences against dirty air

You have these defences all the way from nose to air sacs.

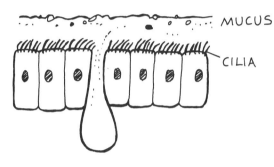

MUCUS

CILIA

1 Don't breathe dusty, smoky air.

2 Tobacco smoke kills cilia.

3 Wear a mask if your job makes dust.

Lymph glands in **pleura** make white blood cells and antibodies which kill germs. You need a good protein-rich diet to keep this defence mechanism in top form. Antibodies are made of protein and so are white blood cells.

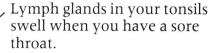

Lymph glands in your tonsils swell when you have a sore throat.
Lymph glands in your neck swell when you have a cold.

If glands in the neck or under the arm swell up so you can feel them and don't go down in two or three days, it is a good idea to visit your doctor.

Exercise lungs and muscles

Old people and people in hospital often don't fill this part of their lungs properly. They can then get **pneumonia** there.

Fling your shoulders back – really work your diaphragm.

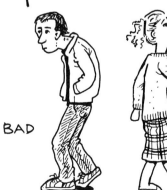

BAD

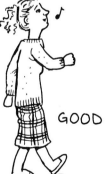

GOOD

Check-up 4 What do you know about your lungs and breathing system?

1 Answer the numbered questions on this diagram of your breathing system.

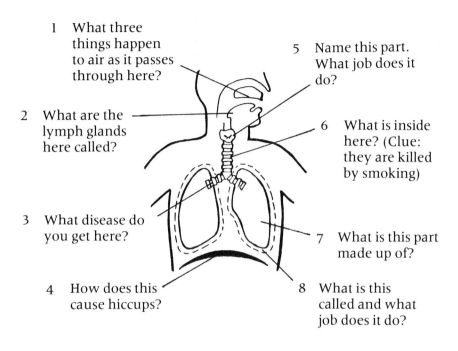

1 What three things happen to air as it passes through here?

2 What are the lymph glands here called?

3 What disease do you get here?

4 How does this cause hiccups?

5 Name this part. What job does it do?

6 What is inside here? (Clue: they are killed by smoking)

7 What is this part made up of?

8 What is this called and what job does it do?

2 (a) These are the five stages for giving the 'kiss of life' but they are all jumbled up. Sort them into their proper order.

- Blow through the mouth; feel ribs rise with other hand.
- Bend head back to open air passages.
- Keep repeating all these every 4–6 seconds.
- Pinch the nose closed so no air escapes here.
- Stop blowing and let air come out; help this if necessary by pressing on the chest.

(b) When might you need to give the 'kiss of life' (3 examples).

(c) What two things might cause a blockage and stop air getting into the lungs? How would you remove these blockages?

3 Make a table like the one below and fill in the missing parts.

Name of disease	Which parts of your body it affects	Treatment
Bronchitis		
Tonsillitis		
Laryngitis		
Sinusitis		

4 (a) In the word search below, find six words to do with your lungs and breathing system.

```
A X C B Y D O P
V E D L Q T R M
L S I N U S E S
V Y A U P F B D
C R P L E U R A
I N H M W Z F K
L A R Y N X G R
I X A Z C N H T
A L G P W R V I
U S M U C U S J
```

(b) For each word that you have found write a sentence containing that word.

5 How many situations can you think of where a mask is needed? (You should be able to think of at least four). For each situation write down why a mask is needed.

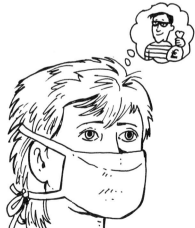

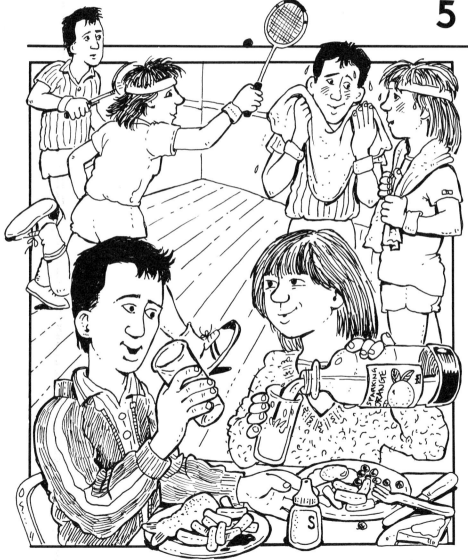

The Salt and Water
5 Balance in Your Body

Losing salt and water

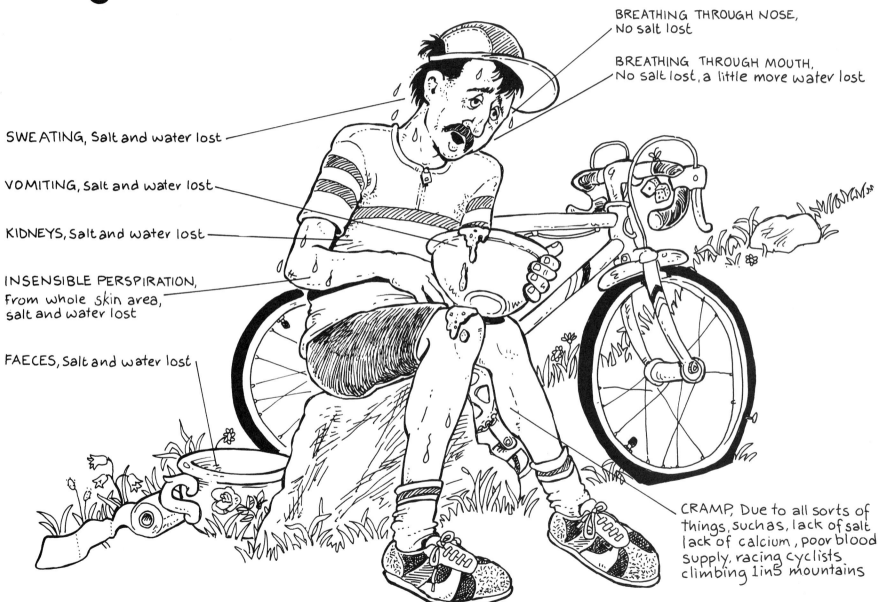

BREATHING THROUGH NOSE, No salt lost

BREATHING THROUGH MOUTH, No salt lost, a little more water lost

SWEATING, Salt and water lost

VOMITING, Salt and water lost

KIDNEYS, Salt and water lost

INSENSIBLE PERSPIRATION, from whole skin area, salt and water lost

FAECES, Salt and water lost

CRAMP, Due to all sorts of things, such as, lack of salt lack of calcium, poor blood supply, racing cyclists climbing 1in5 mountains

Where you lose salt and water

You lose water when you breathe.
The air you breathe out contains water picked up from the moist surface of your lungs (about 400 cm³ each day).

Vomiting
After vomiting you usually feel thirsty. This is because water (and salt) has been lost and the body is dehydrated ('dried out').

Kidneys and bladder
You lose the largest amount of water from your body each day in the urine (about 1500 cm³). Urine contains salt and other substances.

Faeces
You lose about 100 cm³ of water a day in faeces.

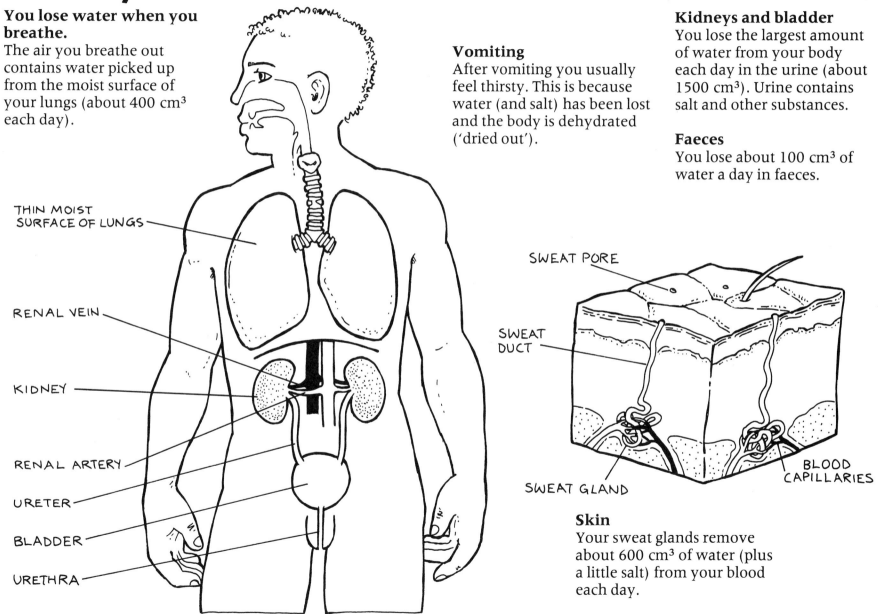

THIN MOIST SURFACE OF LUNGS

RENAL VEIN

KIDNEY

RENAL ARTERY

URETER

BLADDER

URETHRA

SWEAT PORE

SWEAT DUCT

SWEAT GLAND

BLOOD CAPILLARIES

Skin
Your sweat glands remove about 600 cm³ of water (plus a little salt) from your blood each day.

Salt drips

A salt drip goes into your vein. The 'drip' makes
you better quicker.
They are used in hospitals:

1 after losing blood, in an accident or operation

2 after vomiting, heat stroke or burns.

Patients may be too ill to
drink.
The salt (saline) drip is the
same concentration as the
salt in your body fluids, and
it goes straight into your
blood.
If you want to know what it
would taste like, it's about as
salty as you might like your
soup!

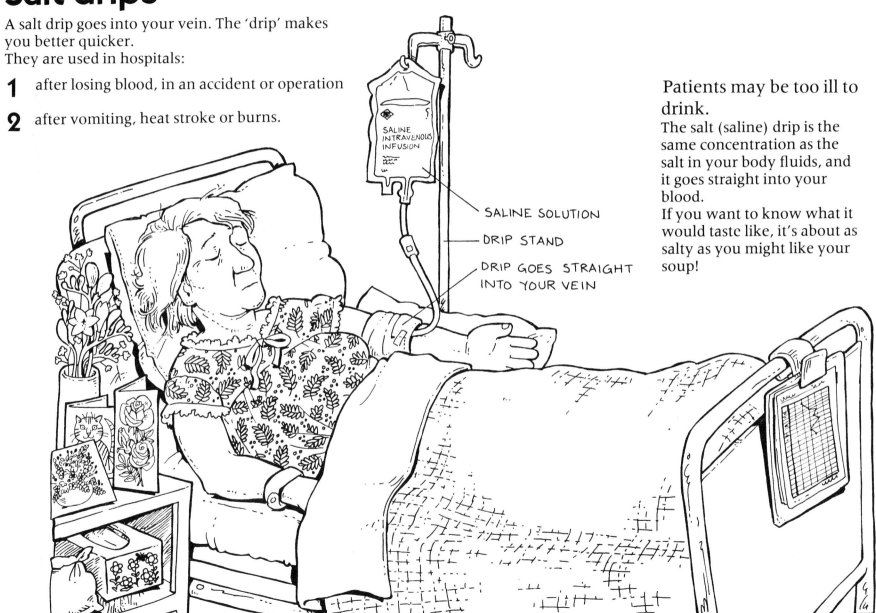

SALINE
INTRAVENOUS
INFUSION

SALINE SOLUTION

DRIP STAND

DRIP GOES STRAIGHT
INTO YOUR VEIN

What happens if...?

Your blood hasn't enough water in it, or is too **concentrated**, or your body is **dehydrated**, or you are lacking salt.

All add up to the same thing – a lack of salt and water.

Your nose
can't take water from your blood to humidify (make damp) the air going in, nor to make mucus to clean it.

Your mouth
can't take water from your blood to make saliva.

Your muscles
feel weak, you feel droopy. You may get cramp.

Your brain and nerves
can't work without salt and potassium.

Your eyes
can't take water from your blood to make tears so they feel sandy or gritty. They can get infected because tears usually clean them.

Your sweat glands
can't take water from your blood to make sweat, so you get hotter and hotter.

Your kidneys
can't take water from your blood to make urine.

How do you lose too much water and salt?

Sweating
Drinking alcohol
Vomiting }
Diarrhoea } especially in babies and toddlers

1 Getting too hot and sweating, then only drinking water.

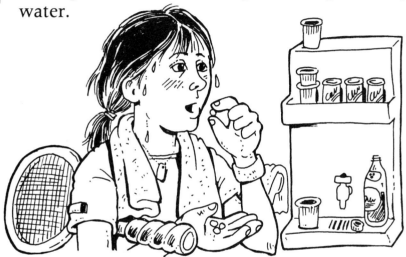

Watch the tennis players at Wimbledon taking their salt pills.

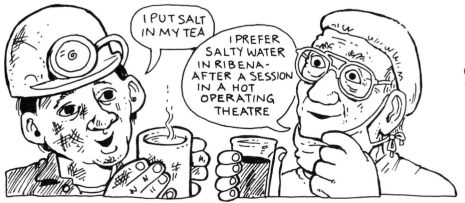

I PUT SALT IN MY TEA

I PREFER SALTY WATER IN RIBENA- AFTER A SESSION IN A HOT OPERATING THEATRE

Ribena has salt in it.

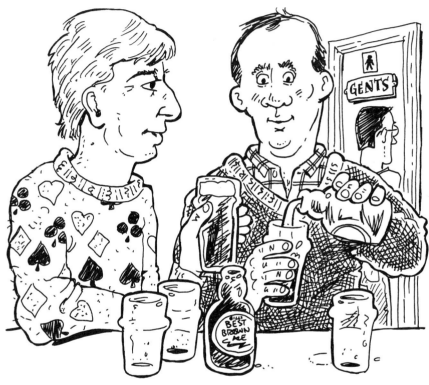

2 Where will they be in 20 minutes time?
Water is taken from the body to dilute the alcohol (a poison) to help it out of the body.
Look back to the symptoms of salt and water lack (page 77).
Many of these are the same as those of a 'hangover' after drinking too much alcohol.

78

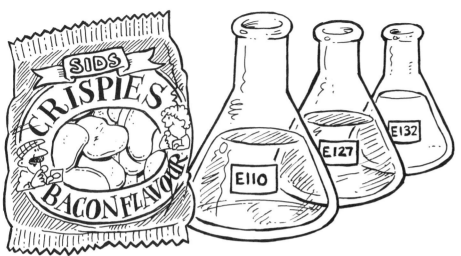

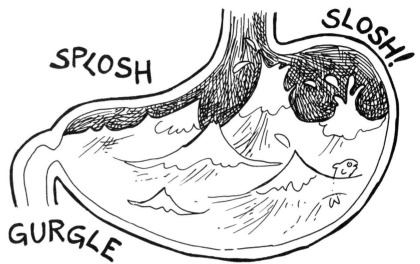

3 Modern food additives
These can cover up the fact that there is not enough salt there.

4 Drinking too much plain water
Just fills your stomach and makes you feel uncomfortable around the waist.

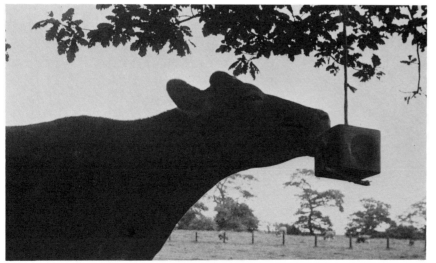

Animals need salt licks, especially in hot countries.

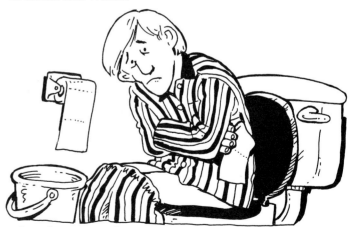

5 Diarrhoea and vomiting
Babies and small children can lose a lot of their body salt and water by diarrhoea and vomiting. See a doctor.

79

Vomiting

How do you make yourself sick? By tickling the back of your throat? Maybe, but **never** drink strong salty water or give it to anyone else to make them sick. Contrary to what many people think, this can be very dangerous. If someone has swallowed a poison, call a doctor or call an ambulance and get them to hospital as quickly as possible.

Most people don't want to make themselves vomit, so what happens when you are sick?

Usually it is your diaphragm's job to enlarge your chest cavity so that air rushes into your lungs – you breathe in.

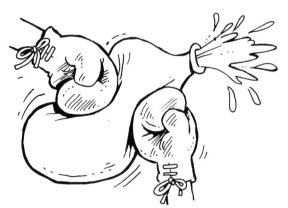

When you are sick your stomach is squeezed hard between your diaphragm and your belly muscles – like punching a balloon full of water between two fists – and out it comes!

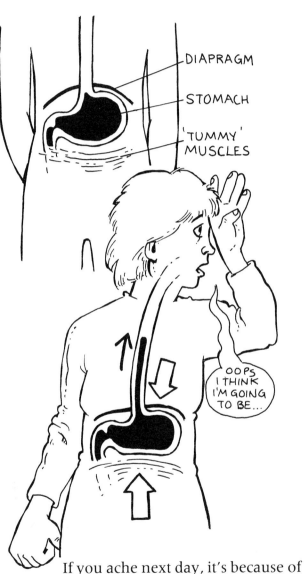

DIAPRAGM

STOMACH

'TUMMY' MUSCLES

OOPS I THINK I'M GOING TO BE...

If you ache next day, it's because of these violent contractions of your muscles.

Maybe you've woken up in hospital to find a tube up your nose? It goes all the way down your windpipe. If you are sick after your anaesthetic it stops vomit going into your lungs and keeps the airway clear. But sometimes doctors put in tubes for other reasons.

By the way, don't use disinfectant to clear up vomit, it smells worse! Use a solution of bicarbonate of soda which neutralizes the acid vomit and takes away the smell.

80

Vomiting is a reflex

It has an automatic nerve circuit which can be triggered off by:

Trains, boats, planes and cars. Eyes and balance organs in the ears are affected.

Nauseating smells.

Solids stuck in the tube going from your throat to your stomach.

Nauseating sights.

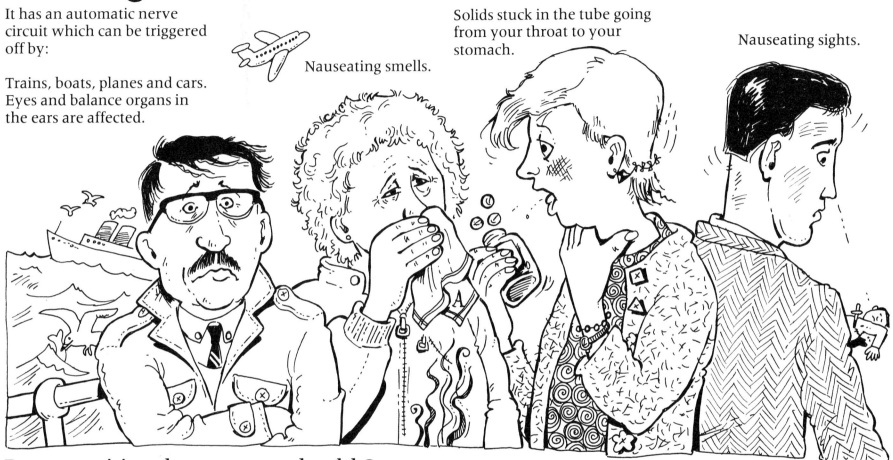

Does vomiting damage your health?

Sometimes it is doing the opposite. It is protecting you by getting rid of food-poisoning germs or indigestible things that could damage the lining of your gut.

People have thought for years that strong contractions of the diaphragm and belly muscles can shift an unwanted baby from the womb. **Not true** – if it does there would probably have been a miscarriage anyhow.

If anyone, particularly a child, vomits for a long time, too much water and too many salts are lost, and the person can get very weak and may get cramps. This is because they need fluids and some salts to replace what has been lost. It is best to see a doctor in such cases.

81

Babies, kids and urine

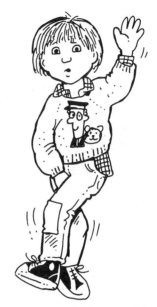

Manages to hold it, until he (or she) gets there – goes 7 or 8 times a day.

Can recognize when bladder needs emptying.

No training needed – when nerves and muscles grow fully it just happens.

Too early 'training' may make later bed-wetters.

Has to keep legs together and dance about if loo is too far away. Bad on visits to stately homes!

Doesn't wet the bed at night.

All babies make urine.

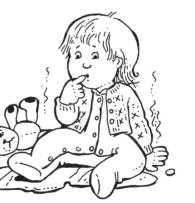

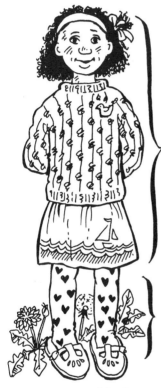

Bed wetters

85 per cent of kids are dry by five years old.

Some take a much longer time, but it's quite normal.

Doctors can help older bed wetters with drugs and there are alarms which wake you before you ruin the sheets!

Making and storing urine

Your kidneys make urine by taking certain substances you don't want out of the blood. It's quite clean here – no germs.

Soreness, burning, itching when getting rid of urine

It's the germs moving in.

They like nylon pants. They make warm damp places for germs to multiply in!

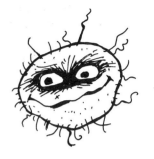

Sometimes kidneys make stones, for example if the blood has too much calcium in it. Kidney stones hurt and need medical attention. Sometimes stones get stuck in the urine tube. This puts you in hospital. If you get a pain on one side only, a temperature and a burning pain as the urine comes out or frequent passing of urine, it may be kidney trouble so see your doctor as soon as possible.

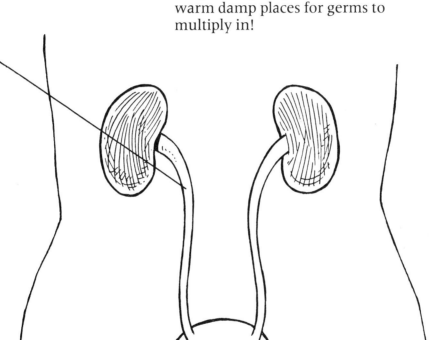

It could be diabetes – germs like sugar too.

Could be you are allergic to soap or talc or a vaginal deodorant if you use one. There's no need to, washing thoroughly is better.

It could be a sexually transmitted disease (STD).

In any case see your doctor.

When you wipe your bottom always do it from front to back. Otherwise you could put germs into your bladder and get cystitis, which is nasty!

Your bladder stores urine and sends a message to your brain when it needs emptying. Don't hold on too long, the bladder is elastic but there is a limit to how much it stretches!

83

Check-up 5 What do you know about your salt and water balance?

1 Copy the table and put a tick in the correct box to show whether you lose salt, water, or both from your body.

When you	Salt	Water
Vomit		
Sweat		
Pass urine		
Pass faeces		
Breathe out		

2 Explain the following and give advice to the person.

(a) When she went to live in a tropical country Kate found she got cramp in her feet.
(b) Carl had a terrific hangover one morning after drinking too much at a party the night before.
(c) Fatima felt very weak, dizzy and hot after a cycle ride on a hot day.
(d) When Jane went to the toilet she felt a burning sensation as she passed urine.

3 Match up these words with the correct description.

(a) Ureter   has sweat glands.
(b) Urethra   part of your body that salt drips go into.
(c) Bladder   muscles cause vomiting.
(d) Kidney   goes from bladder to outside.
(e) Stomach   stores urine.
(f) Vein   makes urine.
(g) Skin   goes from kidneys to bladder.

4 What do you know about your urinary system?
Copy out these sentences and fill in the spaces using the words in the kidneys.

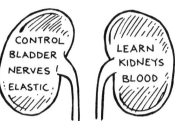

Urine is made in the .... and stored in the .... which has .... walls. Urine contains substances that your body does not want. These have been taken from the ....
Babies cannot .... the emptying of their bladder but as their .... and muscles grow they .... when their bladder needs emptying and how to control the muscles.

5 Copy this outline of the body. Draw in the position of the kidneys, bladder, diaphragm and stomach.

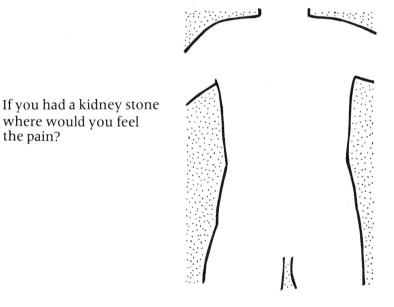

If you had a kidney stone where would you feel the pain?

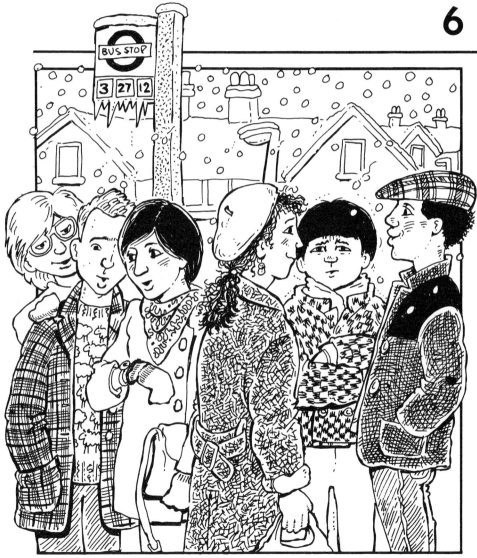

Your Central Heating System

The parts of your heating system

The hairless animal with an undervest of fat.

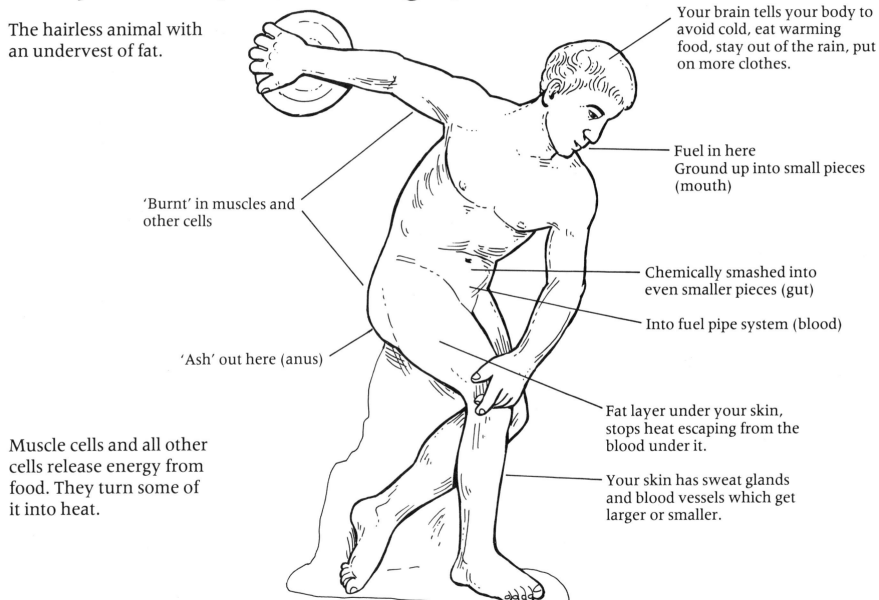

Your brain tells your body to avoid cold, eat warming food, stay out of the rain, put on more clothes.

'Burnt' in muscles and other cells

Fuel in here
Ground up into small pieces (mouth)

Chemically smashed into even smaller pieces (gut)

Into fuel pipe system (blood)

'Ash' out here (anus)

Fat layer under your skin, stops heat escaping from the blood under it.

Muscle cells and all other cells release energy from food. They turn some of it into heat.

Your skin has sweat glands and blood vessels which get larger or smaller.

What runs your central heating system?

Carbohydrates

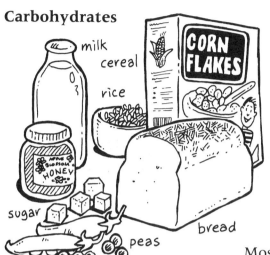

milk
cereal
rice
sugar
peas
bread

Protein

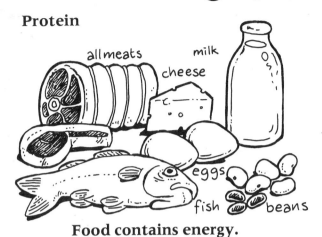

all meats
milk
cheese
eggs
fish
beans

Food contains energy.

Fats

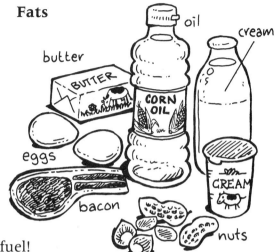

butter
oil
cream
eggs
bacon
nuts

Most of your energy comes from carbohydrates – solid fuel!
But fat contains most energy per gram.

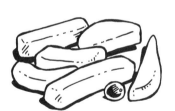

Chips...

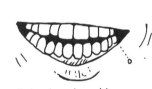

ground up by teeth...

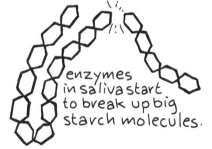

enzymes in saliva start to break up big starch molecules.

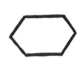

Stomach and intestines finish the job.

All starch smashed into single glucose molecules.

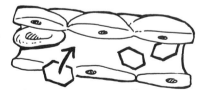

Glucose is small enough to get into the blood stream...

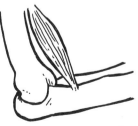

blood takes it to the muscles.

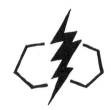

More enzymes smash glucose and release its energy...

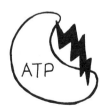

ATP

The energy is stored in ATP.

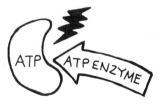

ATP ENZYME

ATP enzyme releases energy to muscles when needed.

87

Feeling hot, feeling cold

Your muscles get hot when they use energy to contract, so exercise keeps you warm.

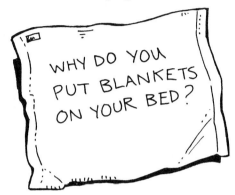

WHY DO YOU PUT BLANKETS ON YOUR BED?

What happens when you are cold?

You shiver

What is shivering? Watch yourself next time it happens. Lots of small muscle contractions. (What will that do?)

The thermostats of your central heating system

They are in your brain and send messages to different parts of your body to

Warm you up

1 Blood vessels in the skin get smaller – heat not lost through the skin – sweat glands make less sweat.

2 Exercise!

3 Put on more clothes to keep body heat in.

4 Have warm food and drink to put heat in.

5 Eat energy-rich foods – suet puds etc. with lots of fat and carbohydrates (but that could make you too fat).

6 Have a warm bath or shower.

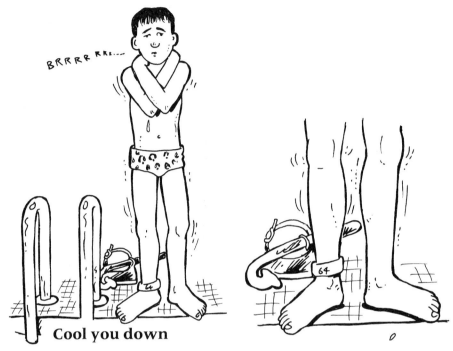

BRRRRRR....

Cool you down

1 Blood vessels in skin get larger – lose heat through skin.

2 Sweat glands make sweat which takes body heat to evaporate it.

3 Move about as little as possible.

4 Eat foods which are low in energy – salads (help to keep you slim too).

5 Take off some clothes to let body heat out.

6 Have cold food and drink.

7 Have a cool bath or shower.

I've got a temperature!

If it's above 63°C (110°F) } You are probably dead or
or below 21°C (70°F) } undergoing low-temperature surgery!

The usual range for body temperatures is 36–37°C (97–99.5°F).

Active children can have body temperatures of 38–39°C (100–102°F). (Don't tell your Mum or you'll never have another day off school!)

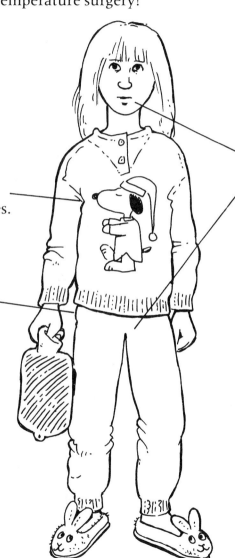

The temperatures of the mouth and groin are usually the same.

Armpit temperatures are usually a degree or so lower than mouth ones.

Temperatures taken in the rectum are usually a degree or so higher than those in the mouth. Why take temperatures of people's rectums anyhow? It's less dangerous and more accurate for newborn babies.

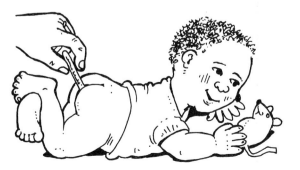

Mouth temperature will be different if you breathe through your mouth – like when you have a cold – or after hot or cold drinks.

Why do nurses take temperatures at 5 o'clock in the morning in hospitals?

Is it because they don't like to see you asleep when they have to be awake and working?
No. It is to make sure they get an accurate reading, before you eat or drink anything.

Taking temperatures

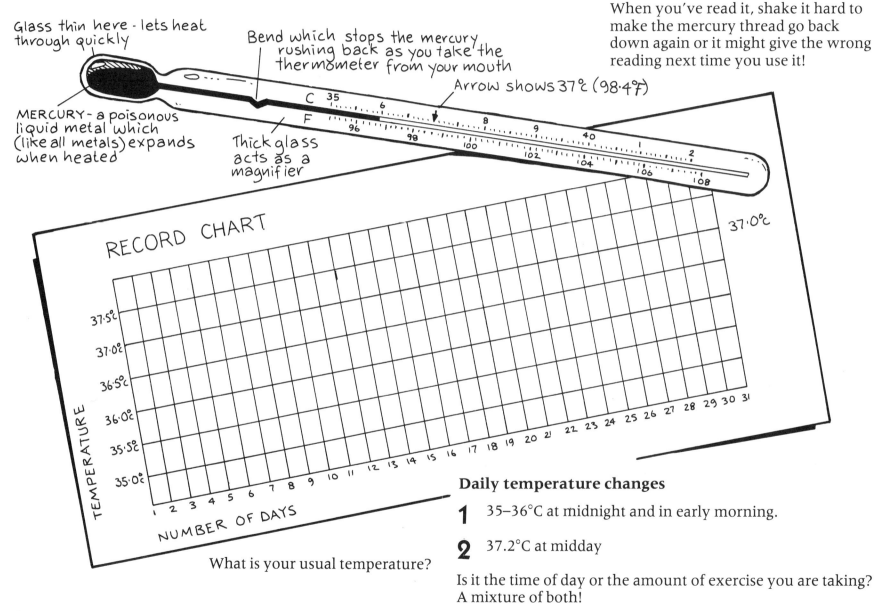

Glass thin here - lets heat through quickly

Bend which stops the mercury rushing back as you take the thermometer from your mouth

When you've read it, shake it hard to make the mercury thread go back down again or it might give the wrong reading next time you use it!

Arrow shows 37°c (98·4°F)

MERCURY - a poisonous liquid metal which (like all metals) expands when heated

Thick glass acts as a magnifier

C 35 6 8 9 40 1 2
F 96 98 100 102 104 106 108

RECORD CHART

37·0°c

TEMPERATURE

37·5°c
37·0°c
36·5°c
36·0°c
35·5°c
35·0°c

1 2 3 4 5 6 7 8 9 10 11 12 13 14 15 16 17 18 19 20 21 22 23 24 25 26 27 28 29 30 31

NUMBER OF DAYS

What is your usual temperature?

Daily temperature changes

1 35–36°C at midnight and in early morning.

2 37.2°C at midday

Is it the time of day or the amount of exercise you are taking? A mixture of both!

What's a normal temperature?

When external air was:	Temperatures taken in various parts of a naked body.	
	23°C	34°C
The temperature inside your 'chemical factory' stays the same.	Rectal	Rectal
		Head Hands Trunk Skin
'Wear a hat or you'll get a cold in your head.' TRUE or FALSE?	Head	
	Trunk	
'Cold hands, warm heart!' TRUE or FALSE?	Skin	
	Hands 29·5°c Feet 25°c	

Range of mouth temperature in normal humans

Hard exercise

Emotion
Hard work
Some normal adults
most active children

Usual normal range

Early morning
cold weather

So there's not much point in taking your temperature just once. Doctors need to know what happens to it when it is taken in the same place at the same time of day for several days. Then it will show if an antibiotic has cured your fever.

Thermostats

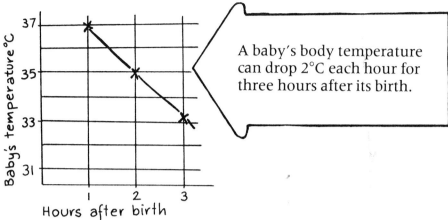

Baby's temperature°C

Hours after birth

A baby's body temperature can drop 2°C each hour for three hours after its birth.

Babies aren't very good at keeping their temperatures around 37°C.

Nor is **anyone under an anaesthetic** or an **old person**. So when you are having an operation the theatre is kept very warm – good for you but a bit tropical for the doctors and nurses!

But why should anyone worry about temperature? Because your body systems work best around 37°C or 98.4°F inside and most people like 20°C or 68°F outside. Old people who cannot afford enough heating in cold winters can die of cold.

Why are maternity hospitals always so warm?
Why should babies be wrapped up as soon as they are born?

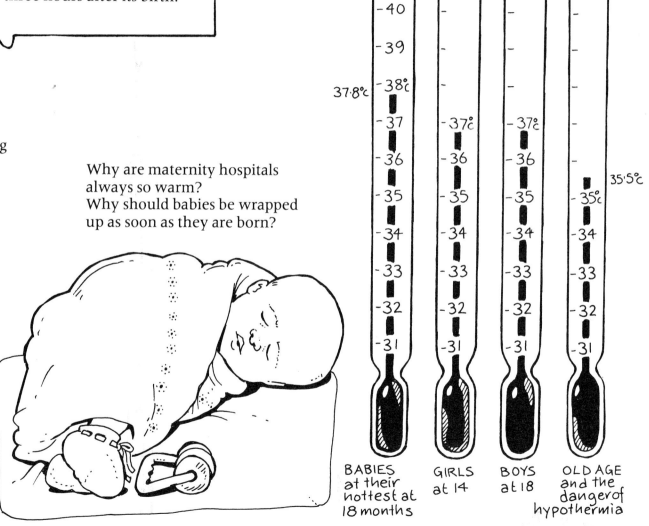

Temperature changes over a lifetime

37·8°c

35·5°c

BABIES at their hottest at 18 months

GIRLS at 14

BOYS at 18

OLD AGE and the danger of hypothermia

92

Human skin

A lifetime of wear!
So look after it!

Keep it clean
But too much washing takes away natural oils and can cause flaking and cracking. Acne is not caused just by lack of washing.

Everyone's skin is different
But most people can't put on weight and then take it off too many times; their skin stops being elastic and sags.

Sun-tan
Looks nice but can increase the chance of skin cancer – it's those ultra-violet rays.

A self-repairing covering which gives protection against:

Ultra-violet rays
Which can be lethal but humans usually just get a tan.

Most chemicals
Don't harm it except when it's cut – then they will hurt.

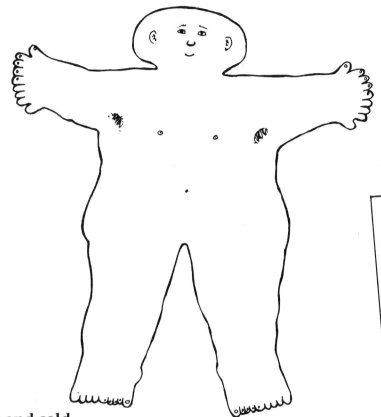

There are 19 350 cm² (3000 sq inches) of skin if you are 1.80 m (5 feet) tall.

Heat and cold
Except frostbite and burns. Never treat a serious burn with 'burn ointment'. Cover it with a clean dry cloth and go to a doctor. The best home treatment for less serious burns is cold water. It takes the heat away.

Water
Skin keeps it in (and out!)

and

Skin is elastic
Can bend into any shape its owner feels up to.

and self-lubricating
With its own dead cells acting like talcum powder. There are 19 350 cm² of it if you're 1.80 m tall.

And your undervest
Under all that skin is your fat layer.
Girls have more than boys. They don't look so knobbly – more rounded curves!

There is not much fat on the head but hair keeps it warm. There is no fat on hands and feet.

Blood hides away under this fat layer in winter, so you lose less heat. You also make less sweat.
In summer, blood comes into blood vessels above the fat layer closer to the skin surface. So you lose more heat and make more sweat.

The gland that launched a thousand deodorants

Man's scent glands used to be sexual signals. Now we wash and put animal scent gland products (that's what expensive perfumes have in them) in their place.

This is where the germs which cause the smell like to live.

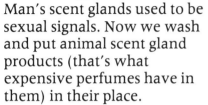

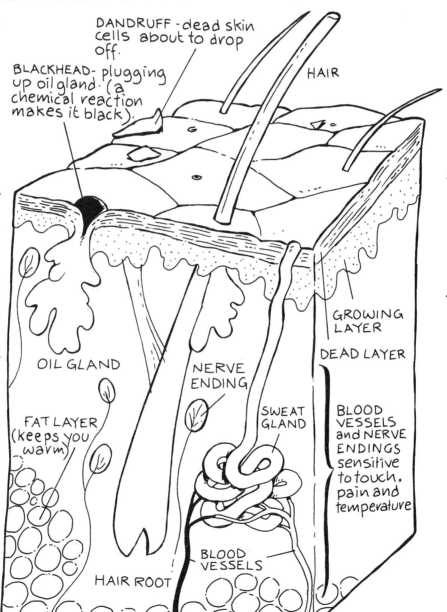

DANDRUFF - dead skin cells about to drop off.

BLACKHEAD - plugging up oil gland. (a chemical reaction makes it black).

HAIR

OIL GLAND

FAT LAYER (keeps you warm)

NERVE ENDING

SWEAT GLAND

GROWING LAYER

DEAD LAYER

BLOOD VESSELS and NERVE ENDINGS sensitive to touch, pain and temperature

HAIR ROOT

BLOOD VESSELS

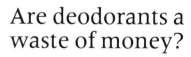

Are deodorants a waste of money?

There is no substitute for cleaning and washing clothes and washing yourself.

Older people don't have such active scent glands – they don't need deodorants like younger people do.

Climate and body temperature

The desert
Pair numbers with letters

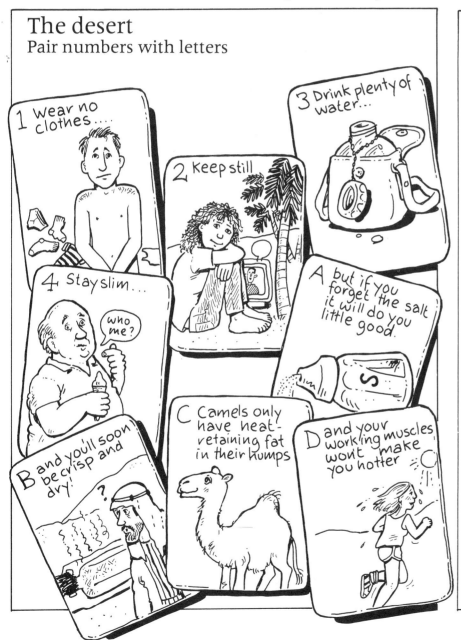

1 Wear no clothes....

2 Keep still

3 Drink plenty of water...

4 Stay slim...
who me?

A but if you forget the salt it will do you little good.

B and you'll soon be crisp and dry!

C Camels only have heat-retaining fat in their humps

D and your working muscles won't make you hotter

Cold and wet
You are more likely to survive if

1 you are fat – keeps heat in the body,

2 you are not tall – less surface area to lose heat from.

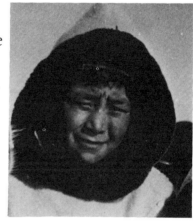

Inuit indians (Eskimos) fit both these rules.

What to do to survive

1 Eat food, hot if possible.

2 Put on more clothes – dinghy sailors should wear wet-suits.

3 Use other humans to warm you – cuddle up.

4 Stop evaporation of water and sweat: get into a big polythene bag – mountain walkers should carry one just in case.

5 Get under a tarpaulin. Wind on wet clothes is a killer whether on mountain or sea. Water takes heat with it when it evaporates.

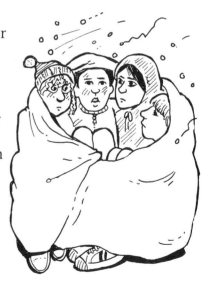

Check-up 6 What do you know about your central heating system?

1 Match up the words in column A with their meanings in column B.

A	B
Mercury	Muscular contractions that produce heat
Deodorant	Skin is this unless it is old
Blackhead	Liquid metal that expands when heated
Sweat	The usual body temperature
Shivering	Chemical that stops you smelling bad
Elastic	Formed when a sweat gland is clogged
37°C	Dead skin cells
Dandruff	Fluid that evaporates and cools you down

2 Fill in the word puzzle using the clues below.
The number of letters in each answer is shown in brackets.

It is a degree or so cooler
than your mouth (6)
Makes sweat for you (5)
Tells your body what to do (5)
When they work you
 get hot (7)
Makes you shiver (4)
Makes you sweat (4)
You can get hot when you
are this (3)
Covers your body (4)

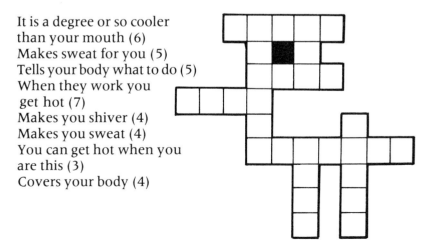

3 When you eat carbohydrates your body gets energy from them which allows your muscles to work. The steps that your body takes are shown below but they are all mixed up. Write them down in the correct order.

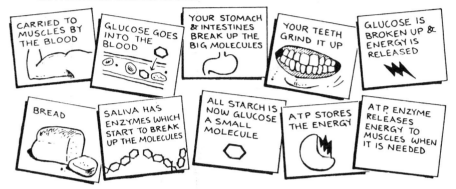

4 Say whether the following sentences are true or false.
For any false sentences write out a correct version.

(a) When you exercise you get hotter.
(b) The usual temperature of your armpit is 37°C.
(c) Newborn babies have their temperature taken in their rectum.
(d) You are usually hotter early in the morning than at midday.
(e) Your temperature is always the same except when you are ill.
(f) Your skin is waterproof.
(g) Shivering warms you up.

5 This man is going out into the desert at 1.00 pm. The temperature will be 43°C (110°F). There are five faults in his clothing. You have to say what is wrong and suggest improvements. Make a table.

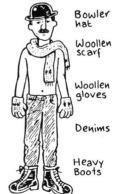

Bowler hat

Woollen scarf

Woollen gloves

Denims

Heavy Boots

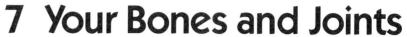

7 Your Bones and Joints

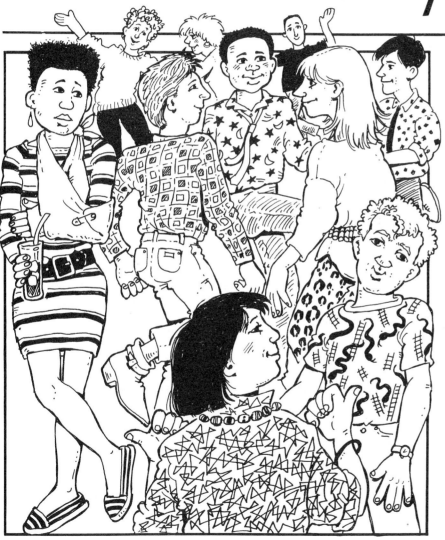

Bones and joints

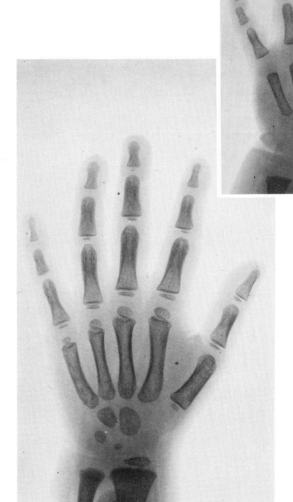

X-ray of infant's hand

X-ray of child's hand

Bones

If you x-ray someone you can see a picture of their bones.

1 All those light parts of the baby's bones are not hard. They are an elastic substance.

2 As the baby gets older, bone gradually forms in the parts that were elastic. Your bones go on growing as you grow, so long as you eat enough: calcium (milk, cheese, cream), fluorine (tap water in some areas), phosphates (fruit and vegetables), vitamin D (butter, fish oils, cheese or lots of sunlight).

3 Finally, parts of your bones nearest the joints change so that they can take the strain, like struts and girders in a bridge.

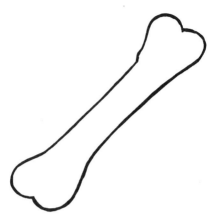

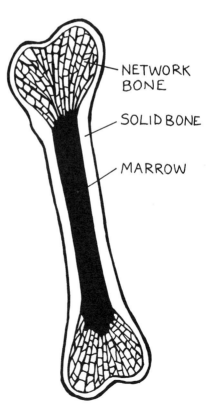

NETWORK BONE

SOLID BONE

MARROW

So you thought bones were dead?

You've been watching too many horror movies

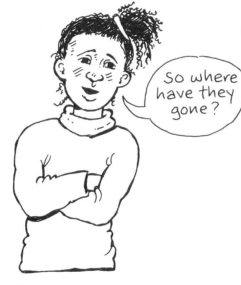

They are living and growing and changing inside you at this very moment.

The bones in you today are not the same ones you had last year.

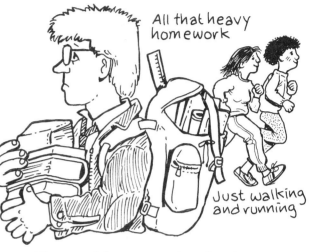

All that heavy homework

Just walking and running

So where have they gone?

The special structure inside a bone allows it to take the strain caused by the things you do.

Bones have nerves too. (You find that out if you break one.)

Fresh bones from the butcher are pink. This is because blood vessels go into them, taking building materials and fuel in and waste out.

Isn't that meat, that pink, not blood vessels?

Yes some of it is, but look for a small hole with a pink tube going straight into the bone. Muscles (meat) are on the outside of the bone.

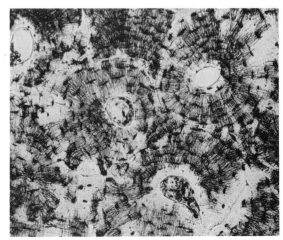

Cross-section through bone

What use are bones?

Their main job is to prevent you collapsing into a heap of jelly!

Bones provide **support** and **protection**.

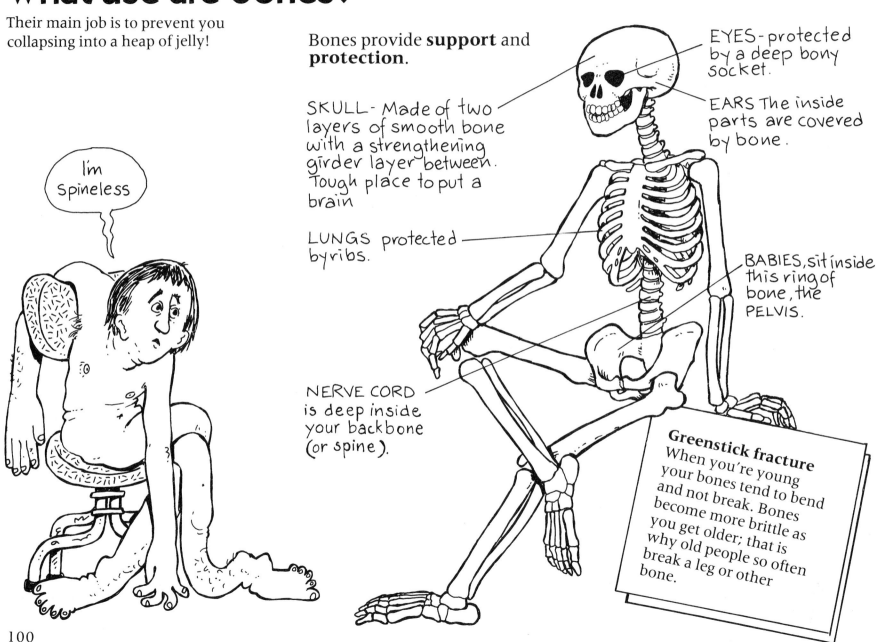

EYES - protected by a deep bony socket.

EARS The inside parts are covered by bone.

SKULL - Made of two layers of smooth bone with a strengthening girder layer between. Tough place to put a brain

LUNGS protected by ribs.

BABIES, sit inside this ring of bone, the PELVIS.

NERVE CORD is deep inside your backbone (or spine).

I'm spineless

Greenstick fracture
When you're young your bones tend to bend and not break. Bones become more brittle as you get older; that is why old people so often break a leg or other bone.

Muscles move bones

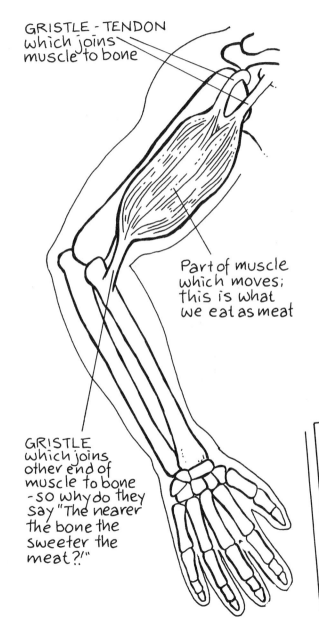

GRISTLE - TENDON which joins muscle to bone

Part of muscle which moves; this is what we eat as meat

GRISTLE which joins other end of muscle to bone - so why do they say "The nearer the bone the sweeter the meat?!"

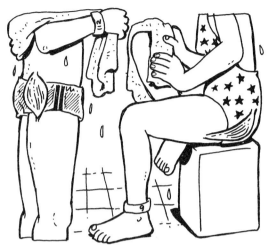

The muscle which keeps you standing! Here it is **contracted** – it is shorter. Now you can sit down! The muscle has **relaxed** (it is longer).

Bones provide attachment for your muscles so that they can move your skeleton. If your muscles weren't joined on to bones you wouldn't be able to move.

And while we're at the butcher's, how can you tell leg of lamb from mutton? Poke inside the bone – is it fatty? Or is it lovely red marrow? Young animals have marrow making red blood cells in their legs, old animals make them only in their breast bone. If the marrow is fat, it's mutton.

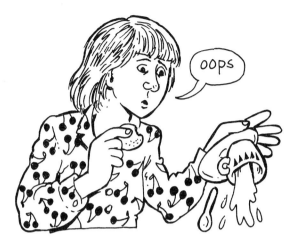

OOPS

As you get bigger, your bones grow before your muscles. Your muscles may not be powerful enough to move your bones without spilling and breaking things, or tripping over things. This makes you feel awkward. Then, in old people, the muscles get smaller again and they have the same problem.

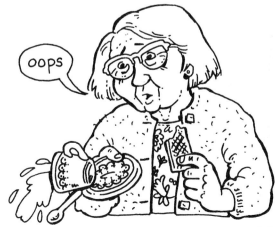

OOPS

Looking at joints

What happens when you rub two bones together? (A horrible grinding noise!)

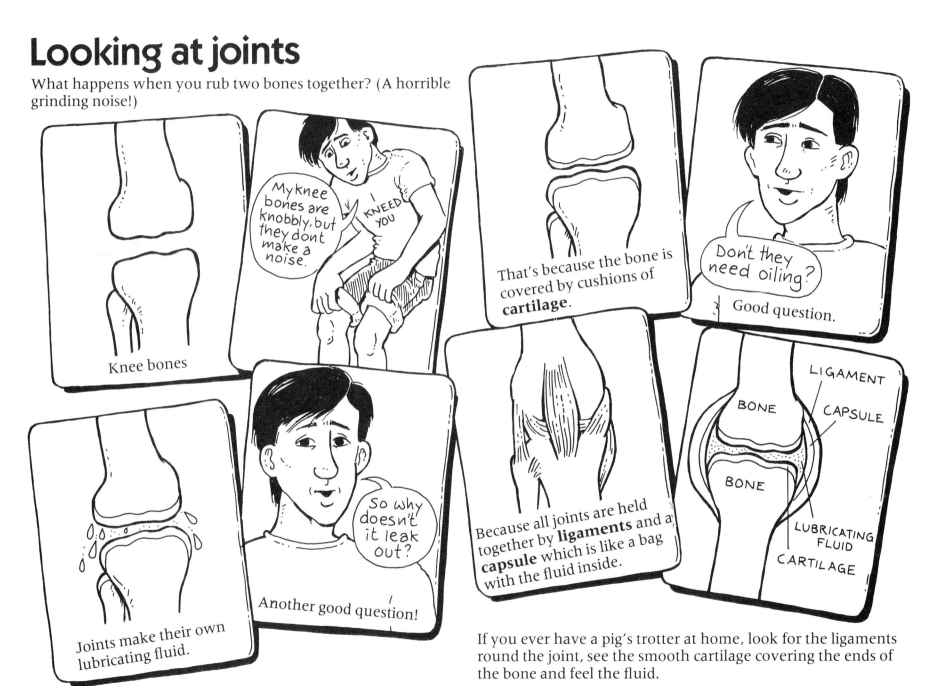

Knee bones

My knee bones are knobbly, but they dont make a noise.

I KNEED YOU

That's because the bone is covered by cushions of **cartilage**.

Don't they need oiling?

Good question.

Joints make their own lubricating fluid.

So why doesn't it leak out?

Another good question!

Because all joints are held together by **ligaments** and a **capsule** which is like a bag with the fluid inside.

LIGAMENT

CAPSULE

BONE

BONE

LUBRICATING FLUID

CARTILAGE

If you ever have a pig's trotter at home, look for the ligaments round the joint, see the smooth cartilage covering the ends of the bone and feel the fluid.

What do footballers do to their cartilages?

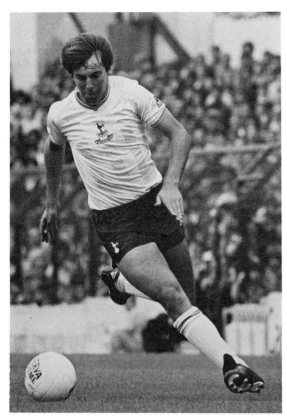

They fall hard on their knees – all thirteen stone of them. (The lightest footballer is about eleven stone.)

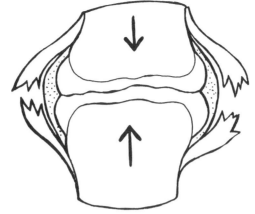

Cartilages can't cushion crashes and the lubricating fluid can only take so much. Ligaments may tear as well. (Only rest repairs torn ligaments.)

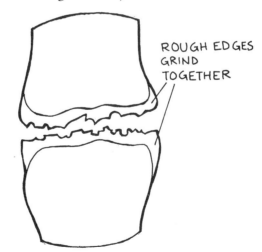

ROUGH EDGES GRIND TOGETHER

Squashed cartilages mean that the knee has no smooth action – it hurts! Removed by a 'cartilage operation'. The bone may be chipped too.

Burst discs

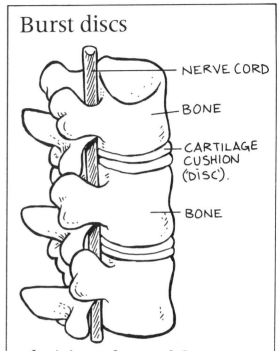

NERVE CORD

BONE

CARTILAGE CUSHION ('DISC').

BONE

The joints of part of the backbone – no ligaments shown

Your backbone has a lot of small joints all the way down. The cartilage cushion between each pair of bones has a tough covering keeping it in shape. Sometimes this bursts and the cartilage presses on the nerve cord – very painful.

This is what people call a 'slipped disc' but it's really a bit of cartilage burst out of its covering.

Torn ligaments and sprains

Where can I tear a ligament? (Maybe it's just a sprain.)
Why do they tear? Because you put too much
strain on a joint.

Tear – very painful – lots of
ligament fibres broken.
Ligament may come apart.
Sprain – painful all the time
– fewer torn fibres than tear.
Strain – painful when you
move in a certain way.

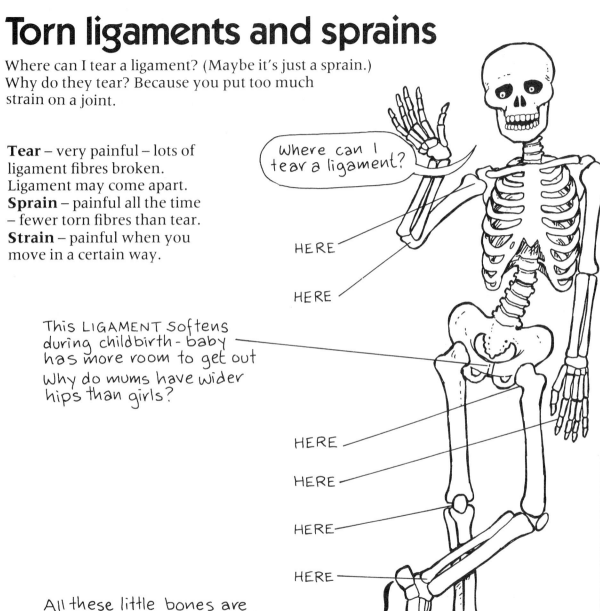

Where can I
tear a ligament?

HERE

HERE

This LIGAMENT softens
during childbirth - baby
has more room to get out
Why do mums have wider
hips than girls?

HERE

HERE

HERE

HERE

All these little bones are
kept together by ligaments

What to do?

For sprains and strains there's
nothing to do except wait, and rest
the affected part. Half a minute in
hot water followed by two minutes
in cold water may help.
If the swelling and pain don't go in
a day or two, an X-ray may be
needed to check there is no minor
fracture. Even if there is, the
treatment is often the same.
Simply rest the affected part. For
pain relief take aspirin or
paracetamol.
Bandage and strap it firmly, and
keep it still until the fibres of the
ligament have grown together
again.

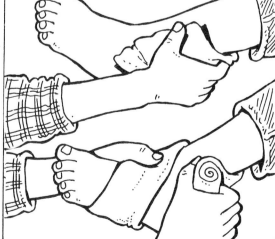

104

Dislocation – putting a joint out of place

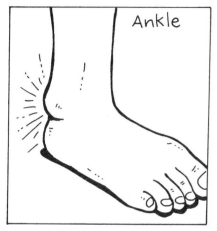

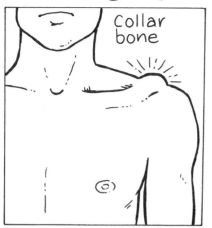

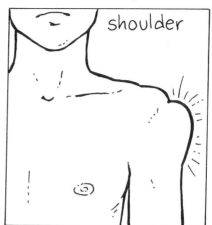

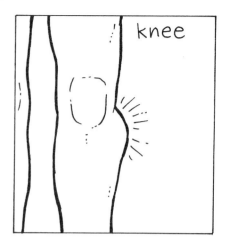

A dislocation needs a doctor.

Keep it still until you get to one. If you try to get it back in place you could damage the cartilage.

Bunions are a kind of dislocation. Often you cause them yourself, but they can also be inherited and you can be born with one.

Don't laugh, they are very painful and can cripple you. Fortunately you can have an operation to straighten the bones again.

Buy your children shoes with straight inner edges.

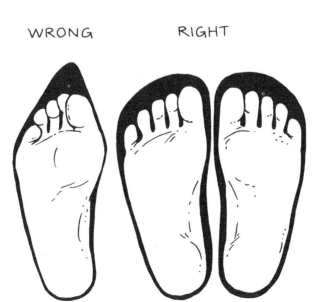

WRONG   RIGHT

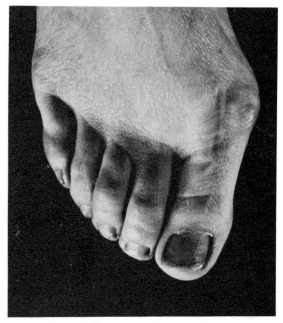

Bunion

Lubrication problems

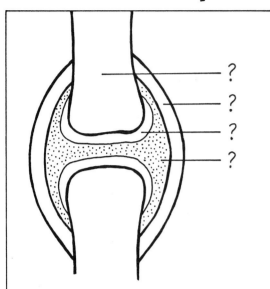

Normal joint
You should know what these are by now. If not, look at page 102.

Housemaid's knee, tennis elbow
Sometimes too much fluid collects in a joint if it is used a lot. Kneeling does it – but we don't hear of prayer knees!

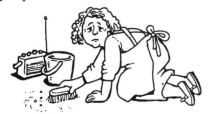

Rheumatoid arthritis

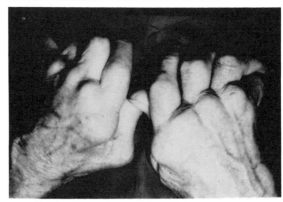

Hand crippled by arthritis

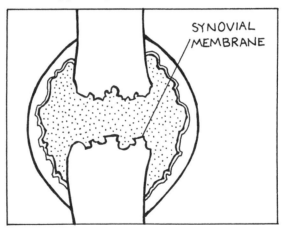

The synovial membrane usually makes the lubricating fluid, but here it has grown right into the bone and the cartilage, and has pushed out the ligament, swelling the joint.

A drug called cortisone can help, but not always.

Osteoarthrosis

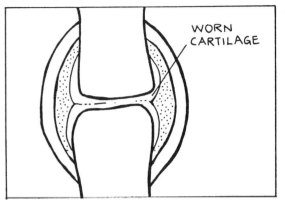

Cartilage is not replaced once it has worn away, so bone grinds on bone.

Joint with gout

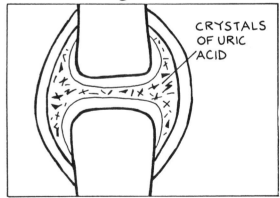

Crystals (of uric acid) grind into the cartilage – very painful.

Gout happens when the body chemistry has gone wrong. There are sharp crystals in the joint's lubricating fluid.

Avoiding backache

When lifting, use your stomach muscles and **keep your back straight**. Bend your knees, not your back.

Weight lifters have a belt to help them keep their stomach muscles tense.

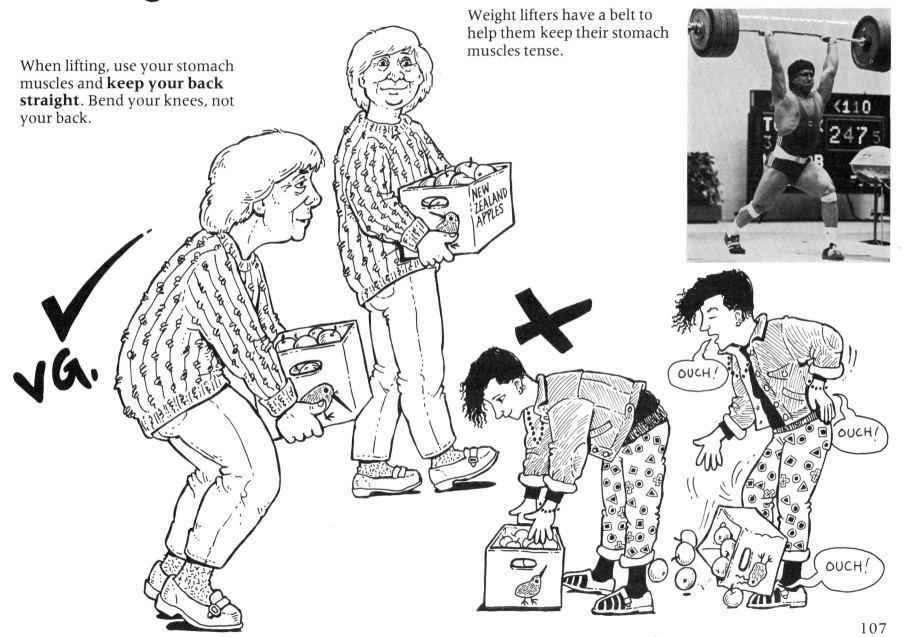

Check-up 7 What do you know about your bones and joints?

1 Look at this picture of a joint. Make a table like the one below and fill it in.

Part number	Name	What does it do?
1 2 3 4 5		

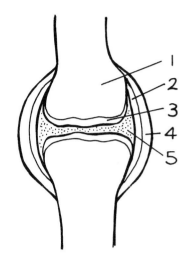

2 These sentences have the words mixed up.
The first word in the sentence is in italic type. Sort out the sentences and write out the correct version.

(a) bones growing *Your* living are and at this inside you right moment.

(b) very they *It* have is a you break because in if nerves painful of bone lots them.

(c) *Your* and to protect bones help your lungs body your other parts of.

(d) older bones your become *When* you get brittle more.

(e) lots of small *Your* made backbone is of bones in a line.

(f) back straight *Keep* heavy your lifting when you are something.

(g) make bones *Muscles* able are to move.

(h) together is painful *Two* very bones rubbing.

(i) found in *Marrow* is the middle of your bones.

(j) pink because *Fresh* they bones are have blood vessels them into going.

3 Write out these sentences using the words in the box to fill the gaps.

tennis rest arthritis pain dislocation spinal cord doctor uric housemaid's cartilages discs ligaments slipped gout

Bones and joints are very important, but things can go wrong leading to .... in the joints.
.... in knees can be squashed by a heavy fall and this means that bending the knee becomes very painful.
.... of cartilage in your backbone can burst and press on the .... in your back. This is very painful and is often called a .... disc.
.... which hold bones together can become torn, again a very painful problem. The only cure for a torn ligament is ....
Sometimes bones can be pulled out of place in an accident. This is called a .... A .... is needed to put the bone back properly. It can happen at the ankle, collar-bone, shoulder or knee. Again, this is very painful if it happens to you.
Other problems with joints are .... knee, ... elbow (which are caused by too much fluid in the joint), ... (caused by crystals of .... acid), rheumatoid .... , osteoarthrosis, and back-ache. All are very painful and you should count yourself lucky if you never suffer from any of them.

4 Imagine that you are a bone in the human body and write a story describing a day in your life.
Your story could begin like this:

'Oh no! Another day in the life of a bone begins. I'm really fed up. My next door neighbour, the thigh bone, has been really squashing against me recently. I think the gristle on the top of my head is wearing away . . .'

Your Muscles and Body
8 Elastic

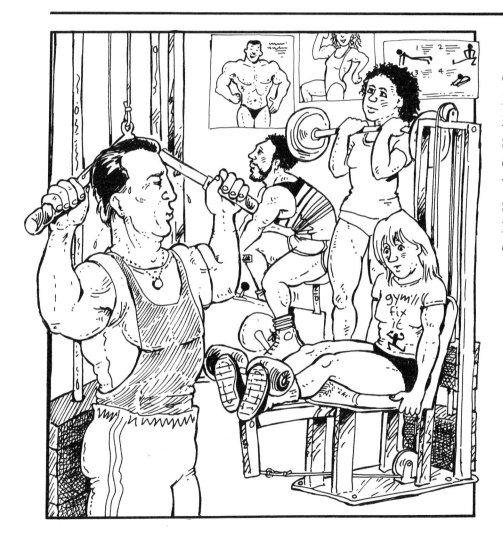

Care and maintenance of muscles

Diet
Muscle is protein, so eating protein helps make muscle.

Exercise
More exercise means more blood goes to your muscles. The blood carries protein, making more muscle.

Muscle tone
In a fit, young person the muscles are always slightly contracted even when not being used (if you are awake). Tummy muscles often sag with age due to reduced muscle, extra fat, maybe harder arteries and general unfitness.

Hormones
Boys have more muscle, girls have more fat.

Anabolic steroids
Your body makes these, but sometimes athletes take extra ones, as a drug, to help their performance. It is against the law. Anabolic steroids build the protein you eat into muscle.

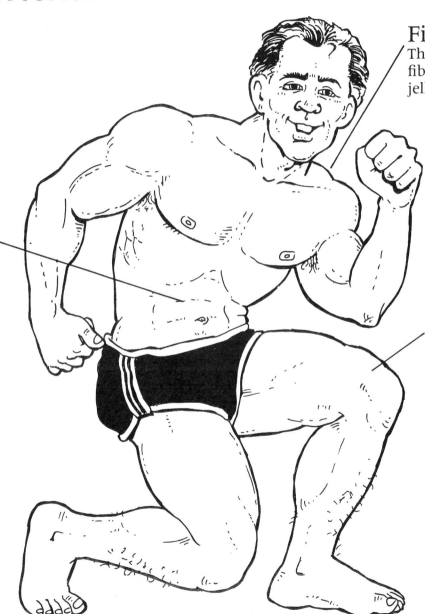

Fibrositis
This is when the muscle fibres stiffen and 'set'. (Like jelly 'sets'.)

Stiffness
A hot bath helps break down the waste products produced by working muscles which cause stiffness. This is why footballers have hot baths or showers.

Tired legs
Caused by too much work and too much standing, so muscles become tired. (Varicose veins may also be caused by these things. The valves in the blood vessels don't work properly.)

Polio
A virus attacks the nerves leading to the muscles; muscles then don't work and waste away.

Movement and heat

Muscles: move bones, and make heat when they move.

Building bits (from protein you have eaten) goes in blood to muscle.

Some protein is used for energy but carbohydrates and fats are used mostly.

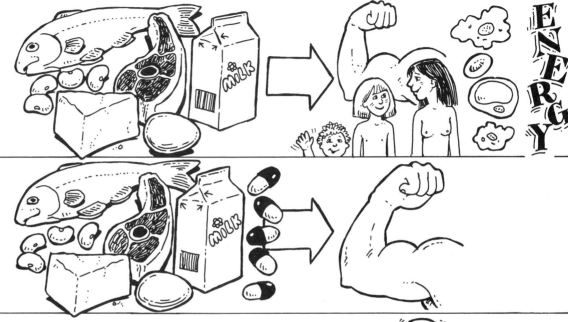

Anabolic steroids
If athletes take extra anabolic steroids all available protein is turned into muscle. None is used to produce energy.

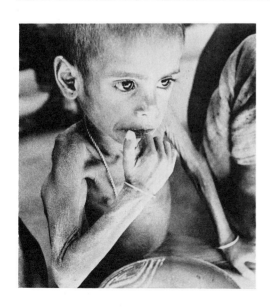

Muscles are not 100 per cent efficient at transferring energy from food to movement – some energy is always lost as heat.

Shivering is when muscles move themselves but not the bones they are attached to. This makes lots of heat and you warm up. But if you have used up nearly all your muscles to make energy, you've very little left to shiver with.

In starvation all protein is used for energy production, even the muscles themselves.

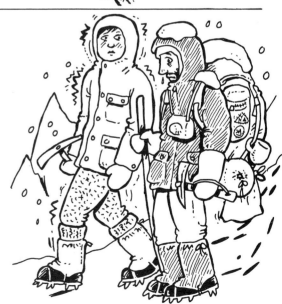

111

Movement makes muscle

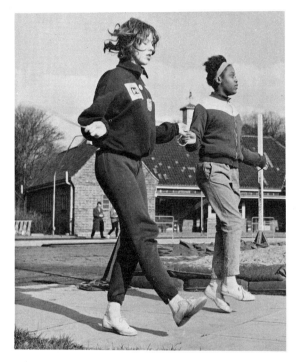

Boxers, athletes, sports people
train using their muscles,
which increases their blood supply,
which increases the amount of building
bits reaching their muscles,
which builds more muscles and blood
vessels.
Some athletes want to build up muscles
faster (or maybe they're lazy) so they
take steroids.

Polio (short for poliomyelitis)

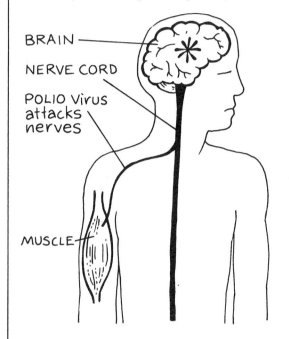

BRAIN

NERVE CORD

POLIO virus
attacks
nerves

MUSCLE

Nerves carry messages from your
brain to your muscles 'telling' them
when and how to move. The polio
virus attacks these nerves.

No message, no movement (paralysis).
The muscle wastes away as it is
not used.

Polio can cripple for life.

Every baby should have
anti-polio vaccine. Every school
child must. Many people have
forgotten, or are too young to
remember, how awful polio is,
so they do not bother with
vaccinations for their children.

(Did *you* have your polio vaccine? It's
given by mouth on a sugar lump, so
doesn't hurt!)

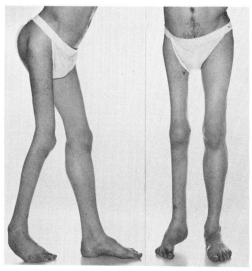

Leg muscles wasted by poliomyelitis

Stiffness, fibrositis

Muscles get their energy for movement from carbohydrates and fats. If they use a lot they make a lot of waste chemicals. If these chemicals stay in your muscles, you'll be stiff next day.

Hot baths switch blood from muscles to skin blood vessels and so clear the waste chemicals from the muscles.

Move it, and a sharp pain spreads down from head to shoulder – fibrositis.

Muscles are like jelly, keep them warm and they 'flow' painlessly, cool them and they set firm.

When you try to move 'set' muscles it hurts!

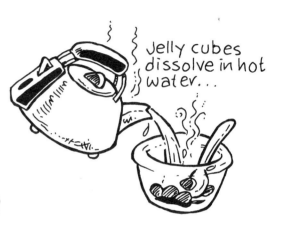

Jelly cubes dissolve in hot water...

When cold they set firm.

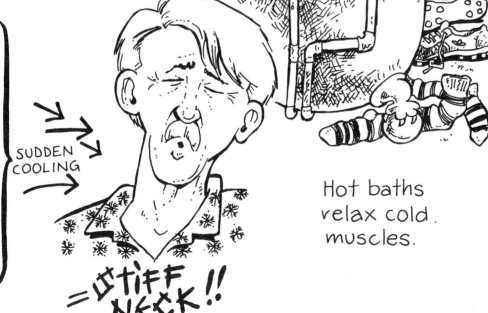

Draughts

No scarf, cold wind

Damp collar

Bed clothes fall off

SUDDEN COOLING

=STIFF NECK!!

Hot baths relax cold muscles.

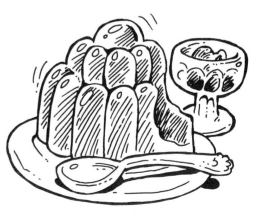

Cramp

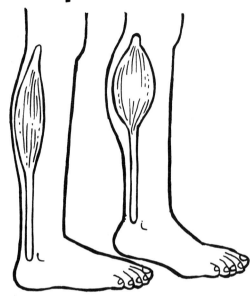

Muscles need

1 Salt You should replace salt lost by sweating during exercise.

2 Calcium } There is usually
Magnesium } enough in a 'good' diet.

3 Energy from food.

4 Good blood supply – to take energy-containing food to them, and to take chemical waste away.

Lack of any of these brings cramp.

Night cramps

You turn over, stretch, then, OUCH, you get cramp in your legs.

1 You will have less cramp if you sleep face down.

2 Less if you have enough calcium (in milk) and magnesium (in cereals and vegetables).

3 Less if you have a good blood supply to your legs during the day. No hard-edged chairs.
Plenty of exercise to remove waste products.
(See varicose veins, page 46).

If all else fails push your heel hard against the floor or the end of the bed.

Night cramps of pregnancy

Baby sits right on top of the blood vessels to your legs.

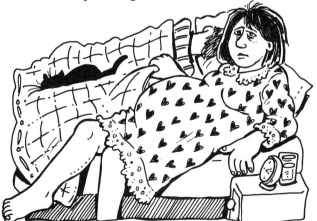

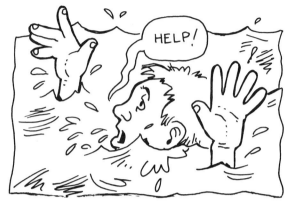

Blood switches from your muscles and brain to your stomach after a meal, so swimming just after you have eaten is not a good idea. Not enough blood to the muscles causes cramp, so you could drown – and it's worse when you're in cold water.

Mountain cycling takes lots of energy and makes lots of waste chemicals. Cramp is a common, painful problem.

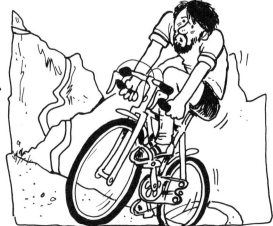

You need stronger elastic!

After forty or more years of pulling against the strain, your elastic begins to stretch out of shape.

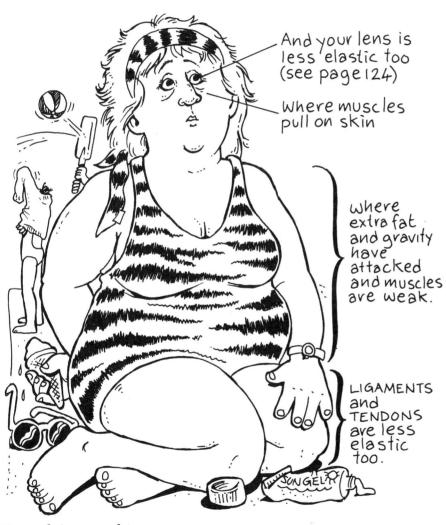

And your lens is less elastic too (see page 124)

Where muscles pull on skin

where extra fat and gravity have attacked and muscles are weak.

LIGAMENTS and TENDONS are less elastic too.

Enough is enough!
(And you may get varicose veins – more sagging elastic. See page 46).

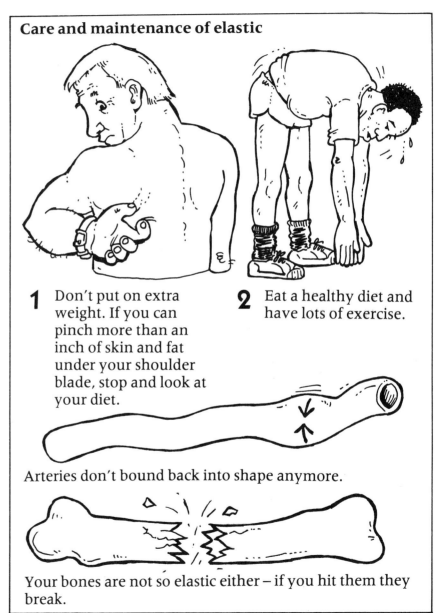

Care and maintenance of elastic

1 Don't put on extra weight. If you can pinch more than an inch of skin and fat under your shoulder blade, stop and look at your diet.

2 Eat a healthy diet and have lots of exercise.

Arteries don't bound back into shape anymore.

Your bones are not so elastic either – if you hit them they break.

Sagging muscle problems

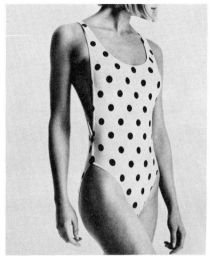

When you're young you keep your tummy in without thinking about it. Your muscles contract slightly all the time – this is muscle tone.

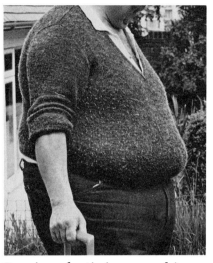

Sagging elastic in your skin, extra fat, lack of exercise and even when you think about it you can't keep your tummy in. Your muscles have lost their tone.

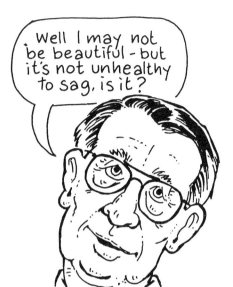

Well, yes it is. If they sag too far you could have a hernia.

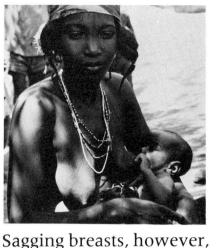

Sagging breasts, however, are quite healthy.

Breasts as long as spaniel's ears still work – but if you don't like the idea, don't burn your bra. Being slim and fit helps too.

What's a hernia?

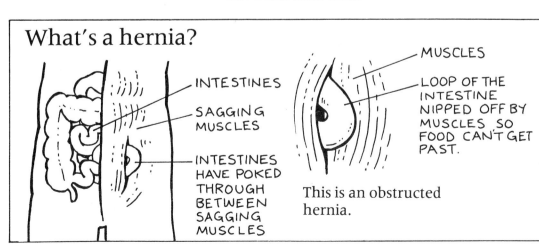

INTESTINES

SAGGING MUSCLES

INTESTINES HAVE POKED THROUGH BETWEEN SAGGING MUSCLES

MUSCLES

LOOP OF THE INTESTINE NIPPED OFF BY MUSCLES SO FOOD CAN'T GET PAST.

This is an obstructed hernia.

Do you have to have an operation?

Most people do. Some hernias can be pushed back in without an operation and kept there, strapped in with something called a truss.

More men than women have hernias because their abdomen walls are thinner.

Human elastic

Human elastic wasn't designed for standing upright, so makers of girdles, bras and elastic stockings make a fortune.

Intestine weight spread out over more muscles, less sag.

No need for bras if you walk on all fours!

Constipation   Faeces don't press on veins and turn them into painful piles (see page 33).

Blood trickles back to the heart more easily – no varicose veins (see page 46).

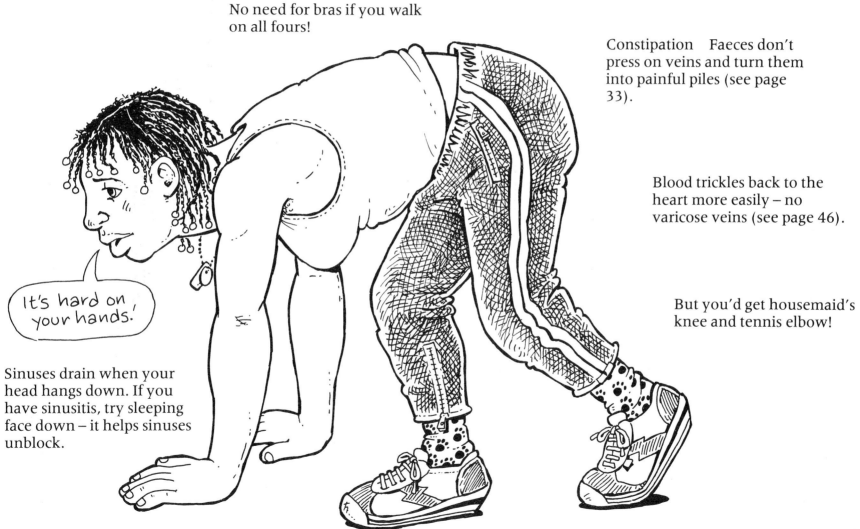

It's hard on your hands!

But you'd get housemaid's knee and tennis elbow!

Sinuses drain when your head hangs down. If you have sinusitis, try sleeping face down – it helps sinuses unblock.

Check-up 8 What do you know about your muscles?

1 Join part A of each sentence to part B opposite, using either the word AND or BECAUSE. Write out the full sentence and check that it makes sense.

Part A
(a) Muscles are made of protein
(b) After exercise you feel warmer
(c) Swimming after a big meal can give you cramp
(d) Losing salt from sweating can give you cramp
(e) Exercise will build up your muscles
(f) A hot bath helps make muscles less stiff
(g) Polio causes paralysis
(h) As you get older your tummy sags more

Part B
they need energy to make them work.
exercise increases the blood supply to the muscles.
a lot of blood goes to the intestines to pick up the food.
sweating cools down your body.
waste chemicals build up in your muscles after exercise.
the heat increases the blood supply to the skin.
the polio virus attacks the nerves going to the muscles.
muscle tone is lost as you get older.

2 When you get older all the parts of your body that contain elastic fibres become less elastic. Write one sentence for each of these parts to explain what changes result from this.

Skin on face   Bones   Arteries
Breasts   Tummy

3 Sally went on a week's skiing holiday. On the second day she found that her legs were very stiff in the morning. Later in the day, when she had been skiing for a while, she felt much better. For the next few days she was still stiff in the morning but by the end of the week she felt OK even in the mornings.

(a) Explain why Sally felt stiff on the second morning.
(b) Why did this get better during the day?
(c) Why was she all right by the end of the week?
(d) What advice would you give to someone who was going skiing to help them avoid getting stiff muscles?

4 Write out these sentences. Use the words in the box to fill the gaps.

warmer	food	energy
exercise	muscle	protein

Muscles are made of .... which comes from the .... we eat.
Muscles need .... to make them work.
.... increases the blood supply to the muscles, makes you .... and builds up more ....

5 Make a table like this one and fill in the answers to the clues. The answers are in the word search below.

Clues	Answers
Drug used to build up muscles	
Muscles moving but not making the bones move	
Muscles need both these minerals (two words)	
Joins muscle to bone	
This vaccine is given on a sugar lump	
Joins bone to bone	
Muscles are made of this	

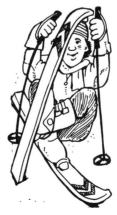

```
E M A G N E S I U M O
D C L Q P E H I O L N
F W B R C C I S T W X
E R L L E S V A C O S
P O L I O T E W R M T
R Z V G D X R X A Q E
O L C A L C I U M Q R
T R D M W K N L P X O
E H R E U Y G W D M I
I V X N U T R Y R P D
N S R T X L E I U O G
B M R N O T E N D O N
```

Your Brain, Senses and Mental Health

9

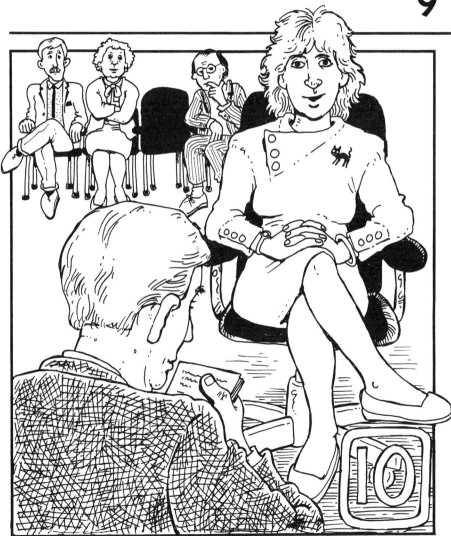

How your brain gets news

to help it decide what action to take.

Your brain gets the largest number of messages from the skin of your hands and feet (but quite a few from your lips – depends who you're with!). As far as your brain knows you should look like this.

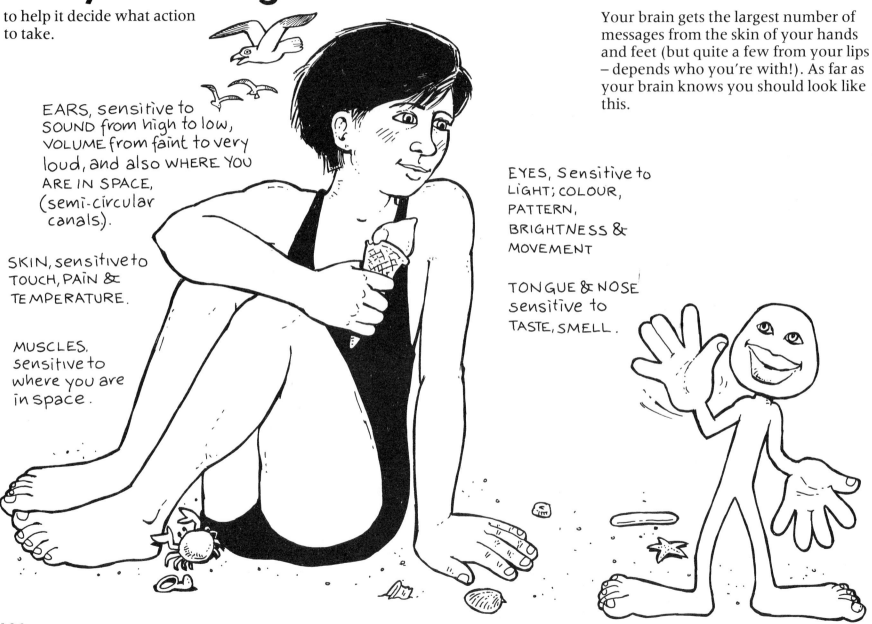

EARS, sensitive to SOUND from high to low, VOLUME from faint to very loud, and also WHERE YOU ARE IN SPACE, (semi-circular canals.).

SKIN, sensitive to TOUCH, PAIN & TEMPERATURE.

MUSCLES, sensitive to where you are in space.

EYES, Sensitive to LIGHT; COLOUR, PATTERN, BRIGHTNESS & MOVEMENT

TONGUE & NOSE sensitive to TASTE, SMELL.

What can go wrong with your brain?

Brain damage

1 Before birth – not properly formed because of hereditary defect, e.g. Down's children.

2 During birth – part of the brain may get damaged, this can cause fits (epilepsy).

3 Road accidents.

Please wear helmets when you are advised to.

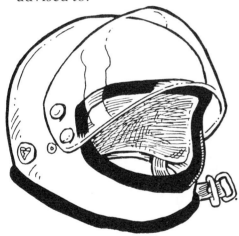

4 Industrial and building site accidents.

5 A growth (tumour) pressing on the brain.

6 Lack of blood – caused by a clot or hardened or broken arteries, e.g. in old age.

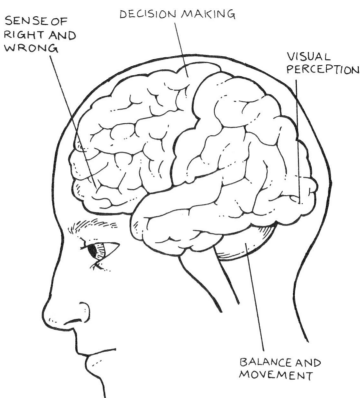

SENSE OF RIGHT AND WRONG

DECISION MAKING

VISUAL PERCEPTION

BALANCE AND MOVEMENT

Infection

1 Of the brain covering, causing meningitis.

2 Of the brain – causing encephalitis (water on the brain).

3 Fevers – scarlet fever can bring delirium, and you often feel depressed after flu.

Stress and strain

- Not enough food, sleep.
- Too much noise.
- Too much to do.
- Not enough to do.
- Loneliness.
- Too many people.
- Too much choice.
- Too little choice.
- Nobody likes me.
- I don't like me.

The list is endless.

Everyone's different. What makes you uptight?

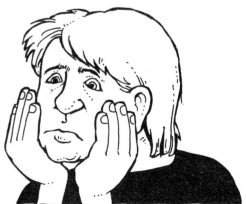

121

Your brain decides what you are going to do

So you think all these arrows are complicated!

It's nothing to what goes on in your brain, even while you're looking at this!

Input   My behind is numb.

Action   OK, move around.

Sorting, using eyes   This page looks complicated, I don't think I'll read it.

Right or wrong check system I think you'd better.

Action   Chew finger nail, read on.

What else is going on in your brain right now?

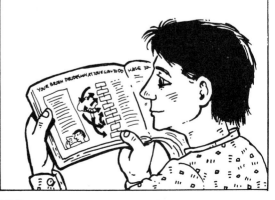

Driving a car

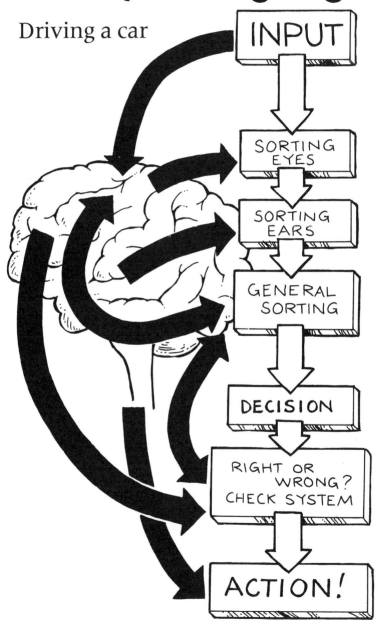

Input   All kinds of messages from muscles, touch-, pain- and temperature-sensing organs in the skin.

Sorting, eyes   What the eyes see: Is that a green traffic light ahead?

Sorting, ears   Where is the sound of that fire engine coming from?

General sorting
1   What did I do when this happened before?
2   Better check that sound again.

Decision   Stop at the traffic lights.

Right or wrong check system: I'd better not go through the lights when a fire engine is coming.

Action   Foot on brake. Action!

Have you ever really looked at your eye?

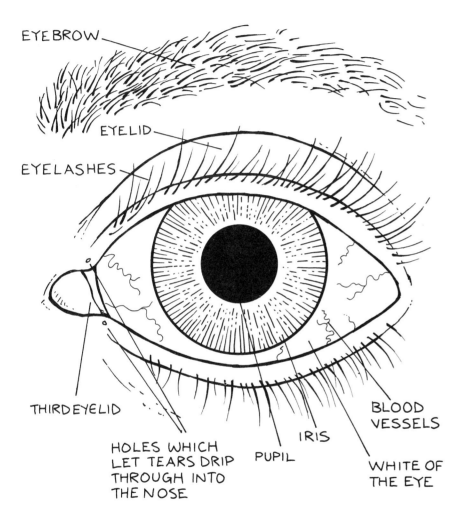

EYEBROW

EYELID

EYELASHES

THIRD EYELID

HOLES WHICH
LET TEARS DRIP
THROUGH INTO
THE NOSE

PUPIL

IRIS

BLOOD
VESSELS

WHITE OF
THE EYE

What use are eyebrows?

Well, they do keep *some* sweat from trickling off your forehead into your eye, but people sweating a lot need a sweat-band.

One boy shaved his off to test this. They grew again but he had dandruff in his eyebrows!

Eyelashes, guard against dust and insects when eyes are half closed – you can still see. The glands at the bottom of each eyelash are sometimes a home for germs.

Iris, the coloured part, changes size of:

Pupil, opens wider in dim light and when you are interested in something or someone!
It's covered by your

Cornea, the 'see-through' front of your eye.

White of the eye, looks pink if your blood vessels are very full!

Third eyelid – that red bit. Not used by us, but watch cats and birds use it as a windscreen wiper.

123

What does your eye consist of?

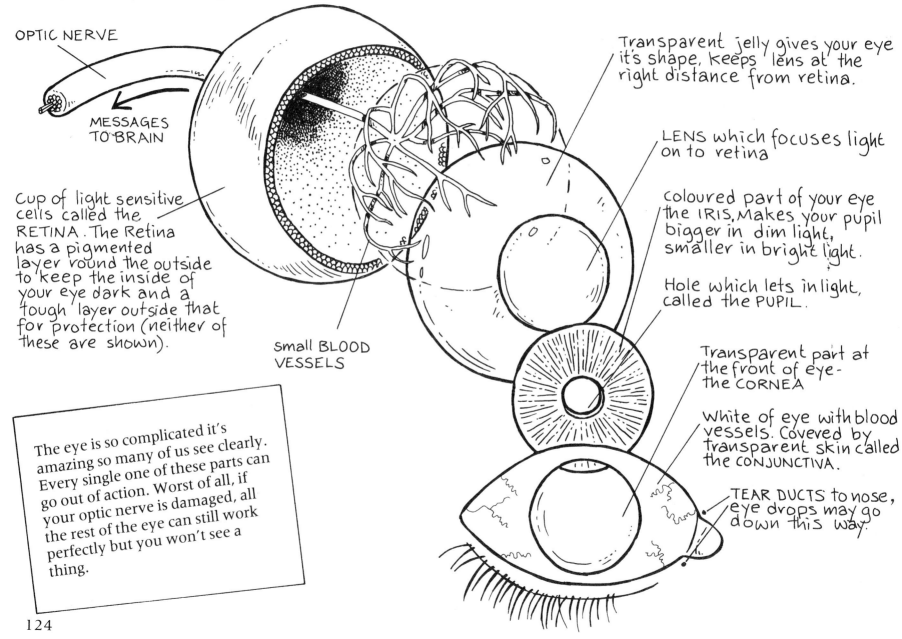

OPTIC NERVE

MESSAGES TO BRAIN

Cup of light sensitive cells called the RETINA. The Retina has a pigmented layer round the outside to keep the inside of your eye dark and a tough layer outside that for protection (neither of these are shown).

Small BLOOD VESSELS

The eye is so complicated it's amazing so many of us see clearly. Every single one of these parts can go out of action. Worst of all, if your optic nerve is damaged, all the rest of the eye can still work perfectly but you won't see a thing.

Transparent jelly gives your eye it's shape, keeps lens at the right distance from retina.

LENS which focuses light on to retina

coloured part of your eye the IRIS, makes your pupil bigger in dim light, smaller in bright light.

Hole which lets in light, called the PUPIL.

Transparent part at the front of eye – the CORNEA

White of eye with blood vessels. Covered by transparent skin called the CONJUNCTIVA.

TEAR DUCTS to nose, eye drops may go down this way.

What can go wrong with your eyes?

1 Retina can peel off – come unstuck – but often doctors can stick it back using laser beams.

2 Small blood vessels can break and let blood out in front of the retina. Laser beams are now used to seal them up.

3 Jelly can have too much water in it and swell up or can lose water and shrink. In either case your eyes go out of focus. If it's serious, drugs can help.

4 When you grow old your lens hardens. You get **long sighted** because your lens cannot focus the light on to your retina any more.

Lens can normally change shape so you can focus what you want to see on your retina.

5 **Cataract** is when your lens is no longer transparent. It can be removed by an operation and very thick glasses used in place of the lens.

6 **Astigmatism** is when your cornea is not curved evenly, so you may, for example, be able to see up-and-down lines better than side-to-side ones.

● Sometimes you can see the blood cells circulating in your own eye (especially if you lie on your back and look up at a blue sky, or when you close your eyes).

● Sometimes you can see a small haemorrhage – looks like a floating fly or tadpole.

● Sometimes you can see spots or even wire netting! Your liver can't cope with your food intake.

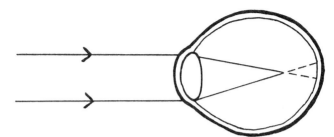

Short sight   Can't focus on distant objects. Can be caused by a long eye – lens focusses light in front of retina.

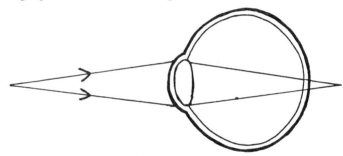

Long sight   Can't focus on near objects. Can be caused by a short eye – lens focusses light behind retina.

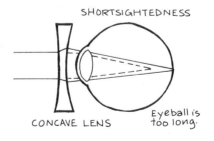

SHORTSIGHTEDNESS

CONCAVE LENS

Eyeball is too long.

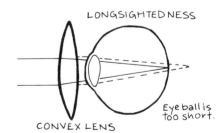

LONGSIGHTEDNESS

CONVEX LENS

Eyeball is too short.

Your skull grows in your teens. Short sight can get worse then.

Your skull shrinks in old age. Short sighted people can often see better then.

125

Never touch your eye

Except with your elbow.

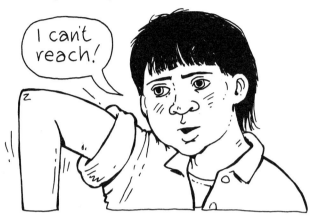

I can't reach!

Yes, well that's the idea – never touch your eye.

But it itches

keep that germ-laden finger away from me!

I'm under your nail

BECAUSE...

The front transparent part of your eye (the conjunctiva, see the diagram on page 124) is very thin and easily scratched and infected (giving you pink eye or conjunctivitis).

You could even break a little blood vessel on the white of your eye if you really tried.

Each eyelash has a gland at its base. Infection here means a stye.

Infection can block the tear ducts.

But I've got something in it!

Calm down and first blow your nose.
This sometimes gets rid of a small piece
of grit.
Grit gets sucked down tear duct when
you blow.
So it didn't work.
Now wash your hands.

No hankies and spit – please!

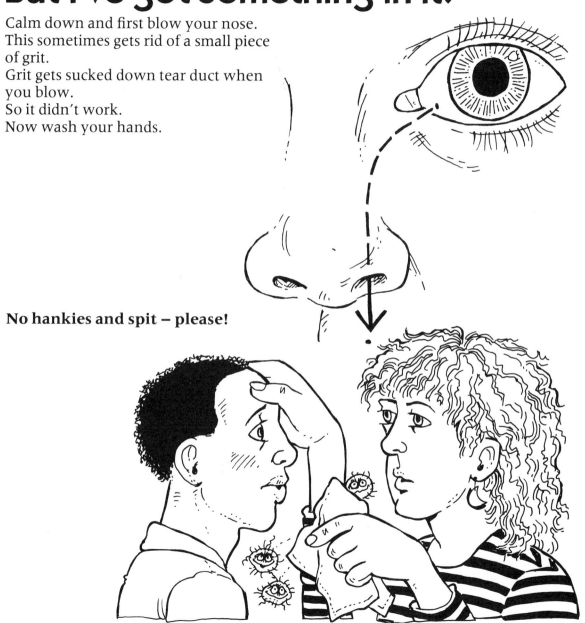

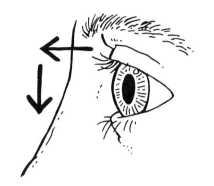

Try this – the best method for
eyelashes in the eye:
— pinch the skin on your eyelid
— pull the lid outwards
— then downwards
— do it again if it hasn't worked
  and once more.

If this doesn't work, cover your
eye with a bandage so it stays still
and no more damage is done. Go to
a doctor.

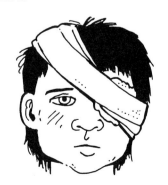

Why do I go deaf when I blow my nose hard?

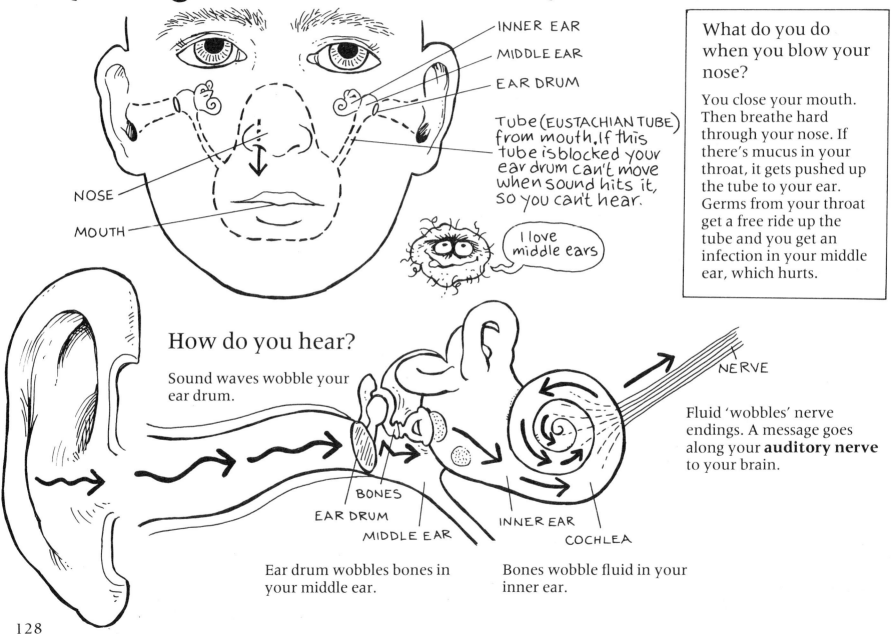

INNER EAR

MIDDLE EAR

EAR DRUM

Tube (EUSTACHIAN TUBE) from mouth. If this tube is blocked your ear drum can't move when sound hits it, so you can't hear.

NOSE

MOUTH

I love middle ears

What do you do when you blow your nose?

You close your mouth. Then breathe hard through your nose. If there's mucus in your throat, it gets pushed up the tube to your ear. Germs from your throat get a free ride up the tube and you get an infection in your middle ear, which hurts.

How do you hear?

Sound waves wobble your ear drum.

NERVE

Fluid 'wobbles' nerve endings. A message goes along your **auditory nerve** to your brain.

BONES

EAR DRUM

MIDDLE EAR

INNER EAR

COCHLEA

Ear drum wobbles bones in your middle ear.

Bones wobble fluid in your inner ear.

Why do my ears pop?

Your ear drum really is like the skin on the top of a drum.

If there's wax on your ear drum, it crackles. If the air pressure is too high (power dives in aircraft, bomb blasts) it can burst.

If your mouth is shut and the air pressure suddenly gets greater, for example

☆ when your train goes into a tunnel,

☆ when your tube train dives deeper underground, or

☆ when your plane lands:

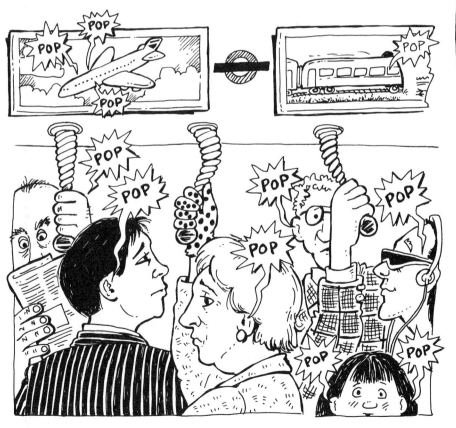

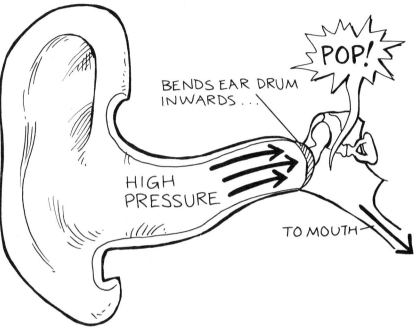

High pressure

Open your mouth or swallow. This makes the pressures on each side of your ear drum equal again.

If the air pressure drops your ears do it too.

When the pressures in the tube from your mouth and in the air outside become unequal, your ear drum bends **outwards**. It happens

★ going up in a plane or up a mountain,

★ in a high speed lift going up, or

★ when the pressure system fails in a plane when it is high up.

129

What can go wrong with your ears?

Wax glands and hairs in the tube to your ear drum usually do a good job. Wax flows gently out of the ears, taking any dust and dirt it has trapped with it – a good self-cleaning mechanism. It also traps insects. Hairs block their way, giving them time to get covered in wax, but not before they drive you mad with their buzzing.

Old wax can get stuck. If you've been diving without a hat or poking at it, it can sit right on your ear drum and make you deaf.

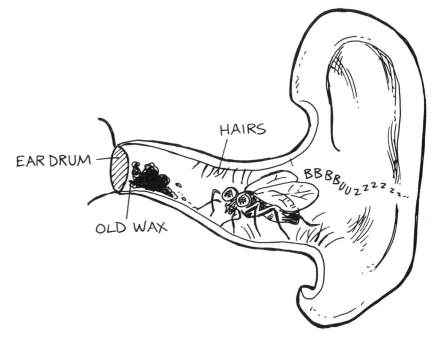

Only doctors can remove old hard wax. Soften it with ear drops before you go. The doctor will squirt warm water into your ear which washes out the wax.

The rest of your ear is inside solid bone – this is doctor's country only!

And, as in the eye, if the nerve is damaged you can't hear a thing, even if the rest of your ear is fine.

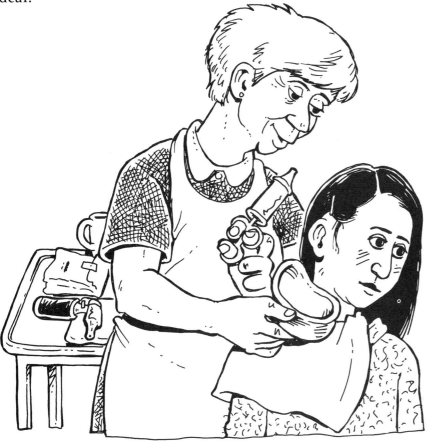

130

Which is worse – being blind or deaf?

(Some people are blind, deaf and dumb.)

Deaf people can see films, read books, watch telly, see sunsets, scenery and faces,
can get around by themselves, can drive,
can lip read, and talk with hand signs.

Find out more from Royal National Institute for the Deaf, 105 Gower Street, London WC1E 6AH.

Blind people can talk to others (deaf people are more solitary, especially in a group of not-deaf people),
can listen to music, plays, talks, tape-recorded books,
need guide dogs or canes and special training to get around by themselves. Can't drive.

Find out more from Royal National Institute for the Blind, 224 Great Portland Street, London W1.

All handicaps mean stress and strain. Especially handicaps of the brain and senses.

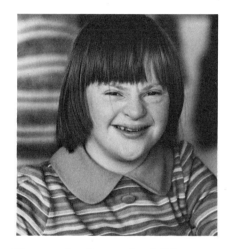

Except for Down's children. They are happy so long as they have someone to look after them and love them.

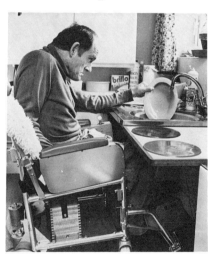

Spastics are people whose minds are normal but who can't control their muscles.

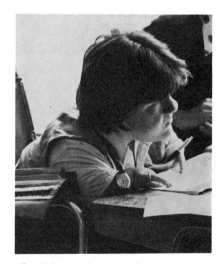

Thalidomide people may have no arms or legs, but their brains and sense organs are OK.

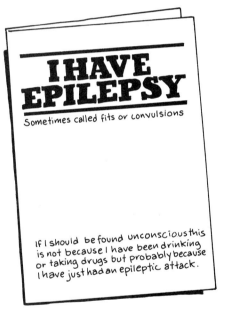

I HAVE EPILEPSY

Sometimes called fits or convulsions

If I should be found unconscious this is not because I have been drinking or taking drugs but probably because I have just had an epileptic attack.

Epileptics (people who have fits) can control the fits well these days with modern drugs. They can drive if they haven't had a fit for three years.

131

Looking after your mind

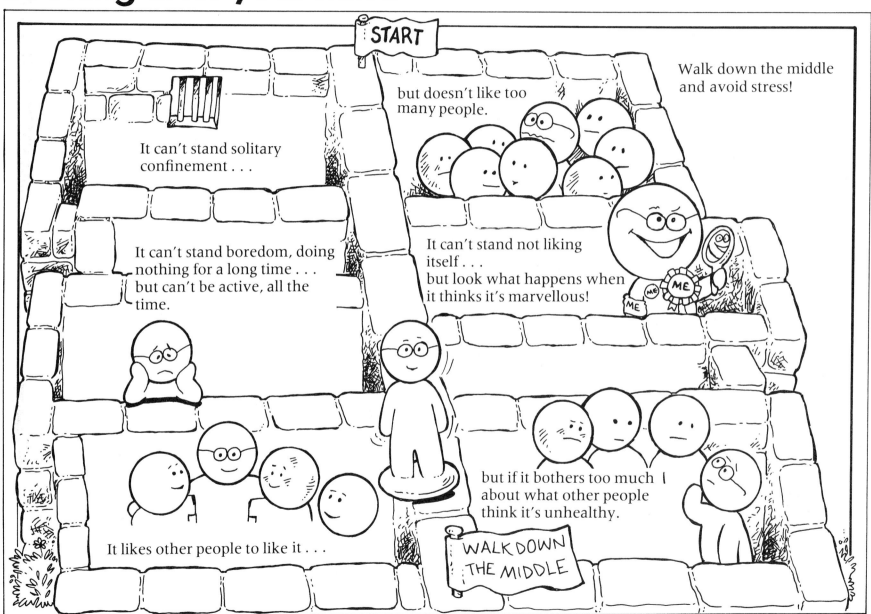

Getting rid of stress and strain

How do you do it?

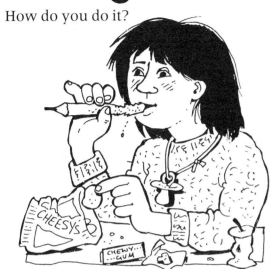

Chewing, sucking, biting.

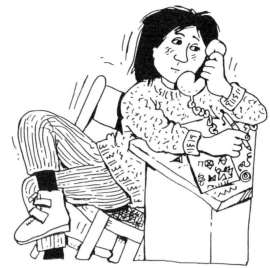

Twitching and fiddling.

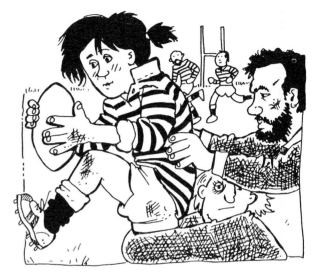

Hitting, kicking, throwing, thumping.

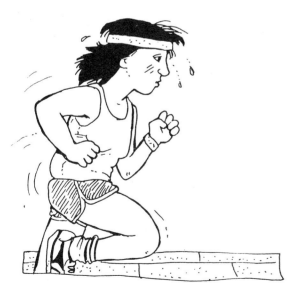

Getting exhausted.

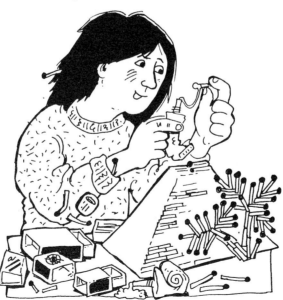

Getting away from it.

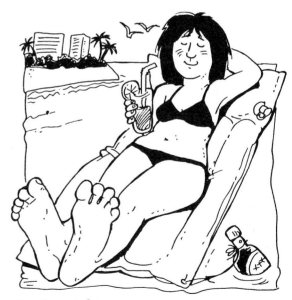

Getting right away.

Brains need sleep

Are you getting enough?

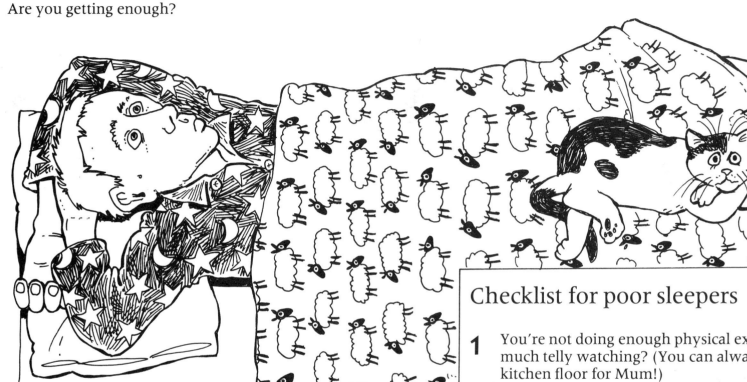

We don't know why. Maybe to sort out everything that happened in the day.

There are two different types of sleep. You go from one to the other alternately through the night.

Dreaming sleep looks tiring. Eyes twitch, snorts, snuffles, bed-clothes kicked off. This is when you dream. You can watch your cat have this sort of sleep too.
The other sort of sleep is much more peaceful to watch. This is deeper sleep, when you are not dreaming.

Checklist for poor sleepers

1 You're not doing enough physical exercise. Too much telly watching? (You can always scrub the kitchen floor for Mum!)

2 You've got out of step – too many lie-ins in the holidays so you go to bed later and later. Break it. Do some hard physical exercise one day and go to bed a bit earlier that night, really tired.

3 Cold, hungry or hot, too full. Your digestion needs a rest too! Find a supper that suits you and don't eat too much within three hours of bedtime.

4 Worried   This makes your muscles tense, you can't relax, and can't go to sleep.

Relaxing

What people use to relax into sleep.

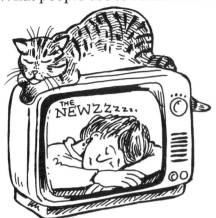

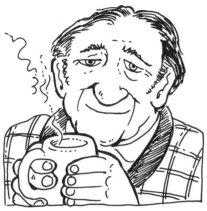

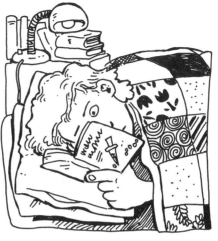

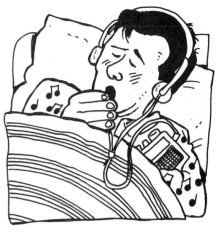

Telly is better than sleeping pills!

In the UK more people use **warm milk** than anything else!

Reading in bed   Shoulders and hands get cold in winter.

Radio   Expensive on batteries if you fall asleep with it on.

Yoga needs practice but it works

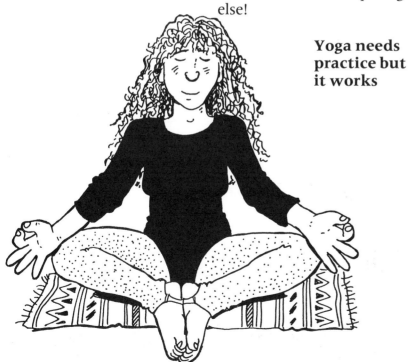

If you don't want to join a yoga class, try this simple exercise.
Breathe in slowly counting to 5, hold it for a second, then out slowly counting to 5, hold it for a second.
Keep this up for ten minutes. Concentrate on the cold air coming into your nose. Try to make your mind a blank. Relax when you get to bed. Check each muscle, roll your head around to make sure your neck muscles have relaxed.

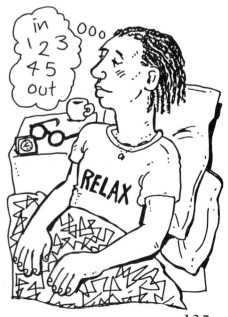

Check-up 9 What do you know about your brain, senses and mental health?

1 As you are walking along the road one day, something happens to make you use your senses and nervous system. Sort out what happens by putting the events in the correct order.

Light hits your retina.
Your optic nerve carries a message to your brain.
Your brain sends a message to the muscles in your arm.
Light from the ball passes through your cornea and pupil.
A girl throws a ball against the wall.
Your arm moves up to protect your face.
Your brain sorts out the message it has received.
The ball rebounds towards you.
The ball hits you on the arm.
Cells on your retina react to light and send off a message.

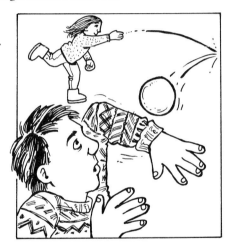

2 Make a list of ten things that cause you stress and strain. Try to think of ways in which you could avoid the stress and strain.
Put your answers in a table like the one below.

Things that cause me stress and strain	What I can do to avoid the problem

3 Say whether these sentences are true or false. For any false sentences write out a correct version.

(a) You can suffer from stress if you do not have enough to do.

(b) Nerve messages travel at 625 m.p.h.

(c) You can get dandruff in your eyebrows.

(d) The retina is the layer on the outside of the eye.

(e) The pupil is a hole.

(f) Blowing your nose can remove dirt from your eye.

(g) Semi-circular canals in your eye help you to balance.

(h) Your brain is working all the time.

(i) Eyebrows keep sweat out of your eyes.

(j) Conjunctivitis is when your lens is no longer transparent.

4 Fill in the word puzzle using the clues below. The number of letters in each answer is given in brackets.

Clues
Eye cover (3)
Layer at the front of your eye (6)
Eyebrows can keep this out of your eyes (5)
Musical instrument in the ear (4)
This nerve carries light messages (5)
Sense organ on the side of your head (3)
This controls it all (5)
Infection of the membrane covering the brain (10)
If the conjunctiva wasn't this you wouldn't be able to see (11)
Your ears do this when the pressure changes (3)

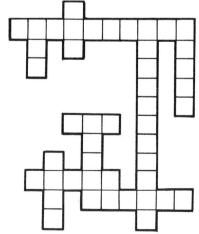

136

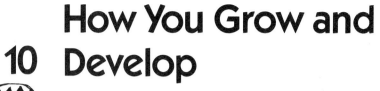

How You Grow and Develop

10

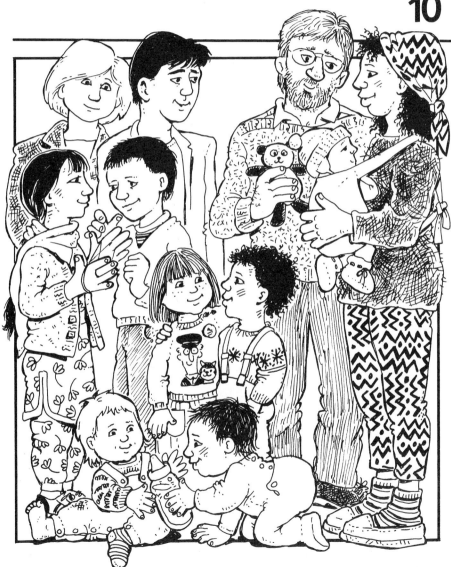

Am I normal?

Whatever your size you get sick and
tired of the same old remarks.
Different parts of your body grow to
adult size at different rates.
You need one size in trousers and
another one in shirts!
And your brain grows last of all.

I'm not normal, I'm the
shortest in the class

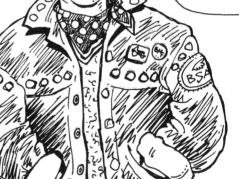

Hello
shorty.

What's the
weather like
up there!!

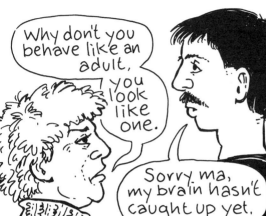

Why don't you
behave like an
adult,
you
look
like
one.

Sorry ma,
my brain hasn't
caught up yet.

Clumsy clots are normal.
It can take your muscles 18 months to
catch up with your bone growth.

So while you are finishing growing
(between 12 and 16) your performance
may drop off in things which need
precise movement and co-ordination.
But it won't last.
Your brain has to get used to using
larger bones and *larger* muscles, as well
as a *larger* view of life.

Child sized muscle
is too weak to move
adult sized bone with
precision.

oops

Growth in height

Your increase in height is really a measure of the growth of your *bones*. Your *muscles* grow later.

Boys
NORMAL RANGE

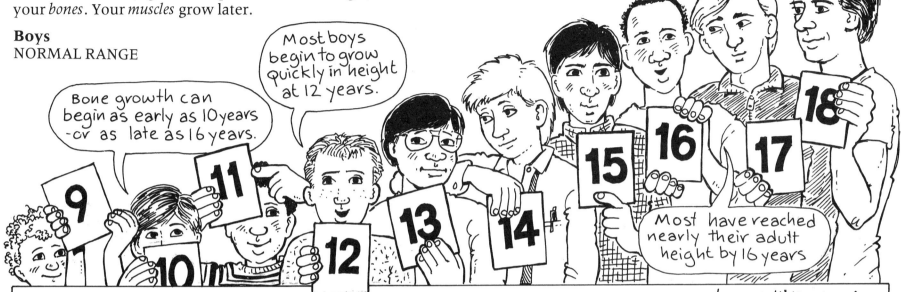

Bone growth can begin as early as 10 years - or as late as 16 years.

Most boys begin to grow quickly in height at 12 years.

Most have reached nearly their adult height by 16 years

Growth is controlled by the **pituitary gland**.
It produces a **hormone** which affects growth.

Very rarely:
Too much growth hormone during the growing phase – a giant.
Too little – a dwarf.

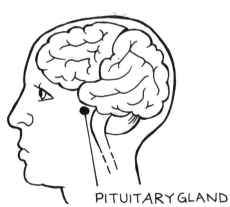

PITUITARY GLAND

An unsolved puzzle: Why do we stop growing as adults when the pituitary gland goes on making growth hormone?

Growth problems are normal

Lots of people end up with one foot bigger than the other and very few shoe shops stock shoes in odd pairs! Growth of muscles, bones, skin, etc. is such a complicated process that it's a wonder anyone is normal at all.

It would be abnormal to be normal, or even average, in everything.

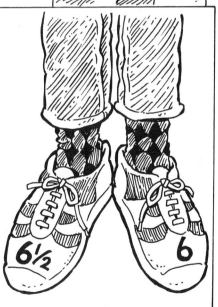

Girls and boys grow at different rates

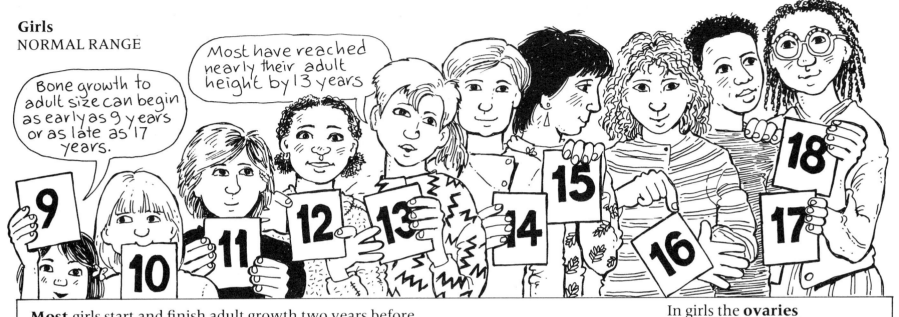

Girls
NORMAL RANGE

Bone growth to adult size can begin as early as 9 years or as late as 17 years.

Most have reached nearly their adult height by 13 years

9 10 11 12 13 14 15 16 17 18

Most girls start and finish adult growth two years before **most** boys.

But boys catch up; one boy who was 4' 6" (or 1.35 m) in the sixth form ended up as 5' 11" (or 1.80 m).

Other measurements vary between boys and girls

On average, girls have wider hips than boys.
Is this true in your class?

On average, boys have broader shoulders than girls.
But in a mixed class there will always be some girls whose shoulders are broader than some boys' shoulders and some boys with hips broader than some girls' hips.

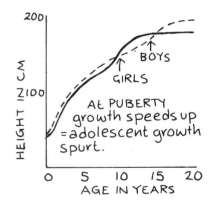

200

HEIGHT IN CM

BOYS

GIRLS

At PUBERTY growth speeds up = adolescent growth spurt.

100

0 5 10 15 20
AGE IN YEARS

These differences are due to two hormones produced by the **sex glands** which affect growth.

In girls the **ovaries** produce **oestrogen**.

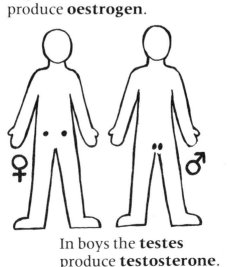

In boys the **testes** produce **testosterone**.

Human variation

How we inherit characteristics from our parents

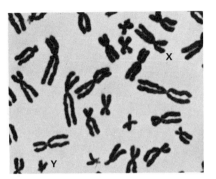

Male chromosomes

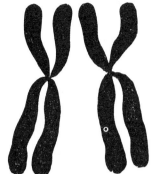

One chromosome pair

Each cell in the body contains 46 **chromosomes**.
Each pair of chromosomes is made up of parts called **genes** which control the development of characteristics like eye colour.

There are 22 matched pairs. The two sex chromosomes are different from each other. When eggs or sperm are produced in the body, they each receive 23 chromosomes, one from each pair and one sex chromosome.

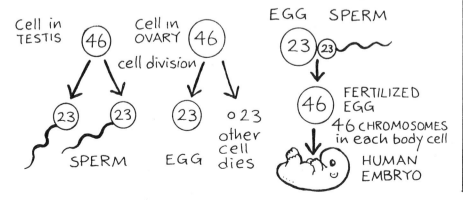

Eye colour

Whether our eyes are blue or brown is decided by a **gene pair**. The gene can be of two slightly different types.

Father and mother with brown eyes.

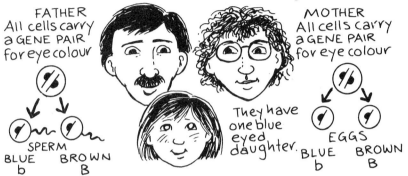

So one gene of the pair in the cells of both parents must be for blue eyes and the other one must be for brown eyes.

Here are the four daughters:

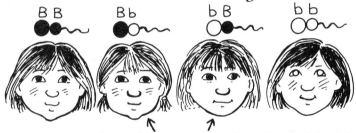

These two girls have brown eyes. The effect of the blue gene is hidden by the brown gene.
The gene controlling the development of brown eyes is **dominant** to the gene for blue eyes.
Some characteristics which we inherit from our parents may be dominant to others. For example freckles, dimples and cleft chin are all dominant characteristics.

Heredity and environment

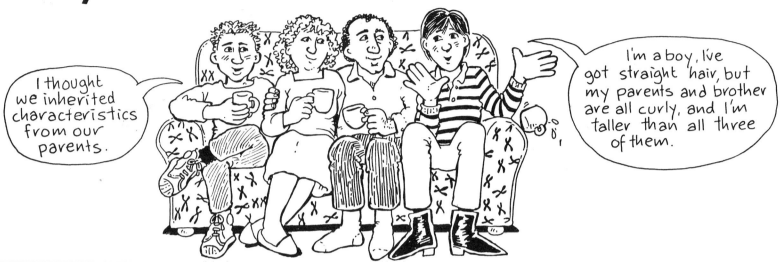

I thought we inherited characteristics from our parents.

I'm a boy, I've got straight hair, but my parents and brother are all curly, and I'm taller than all three of them.

What about identical twins?

They will always be the same sex and often look identical even if they are brought up separately.

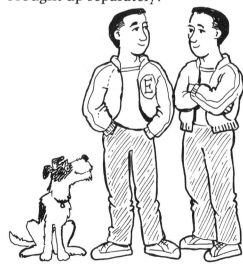

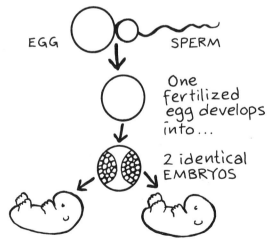

EGG   SPERM

One fertilized egg develops into...

2 identical EMBRYOS

Their genes are identical because the twins come from one egg which split into two after fertilization.

American twins, Edwin and Fred, were separated in infancy and met again aged 25 years:

They looked identical.
They were both right-handed.
They were both repair men in different branches of the same telephone company.
They married similar women in the same year.
Each had a baby son.
Each owned a fox terrier, which they both called by the same name, Trixie.

Heredity or environment?

Differences between people are inherited, but they can also be affected by environment.

Hair

Curly hair is dominant to straight hair.
(See page 141.)

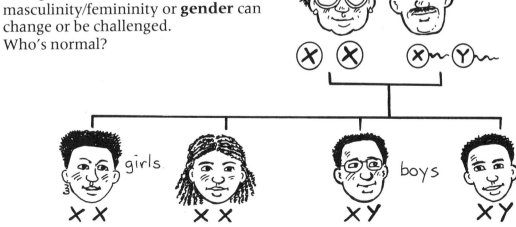

GENES

GENES

Sex

Biological sex is fixed, but ideas about masculinity/femininity or **gender** can change or be challenged.
Who's normal?

girls

boys

X X   X X   X Y   X Y

Height

This is affected by a large number of genes, but shortness tends to be dominant to tallness. Therefore tall parents tend to have tall children but short parents can have children of all heights.

Boys of the same age:

Difference due to better diet these days.

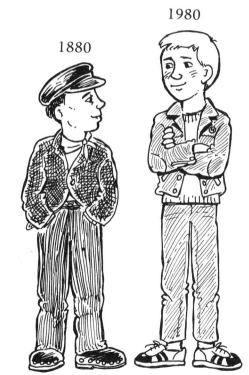

1980

1880

All our characteristics depend on how the environment affects what we inherit.

Fulfilling human needs

All human beings need

1 Physical security

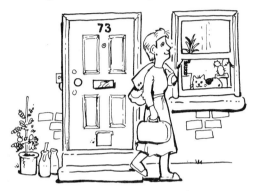

Not to feel hunger, pain, thirst, too cold, too hot, tired.
To satisfy these needs you have to find food, water, somewhere sheltered, and to take care of yourself.
For most of us this means earning a living by having a job.

2 To be respected by others

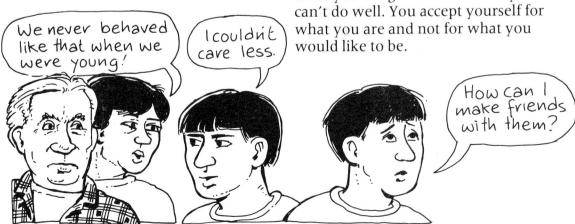

3 To respect yourself

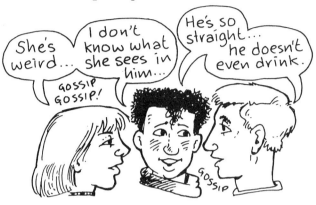

Everyone needs these three.
Maybe you don't care as much as your parents do about what other people say about you, but most people care what people of the same age think about them.

So nobody understands you, but you do understand yourself. You know what you are good at and what you can't do well. You accept yourself for what you are and not for what you would like to be.

4 To mate

Does everyone need to mate?

Does everyone need to mate all their lives?

Does mating mean the same to everyone?

Some people have five husbands or twenty wives.

Some people have one husband or wife early in life and then continue alone.

Some people just think of the actual mating, others are very keen to have its results, babies.

Some use their mating successes as a means of gaining self respect or the respect of others.

You could call it parental care, but it doesn't mean just caring for children, but for almost any person who needs your help.

Doctors, nurses and teachers often have a strong need to care for others, even if it means hard work for themselves.

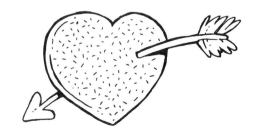

What are your most important needs?

5 To care for others

Teenagers are often surprised to find what a kick they get out of helping the old and the handicapped.

Some feel that the rewards for caring are more satisfying than money.

But some people are just meddling busybodies.

And some are so busy caring for others that they forget about themselves, their children, their old people.

Do you know anyone who doesn't care for someone else?

Is he/she happy?

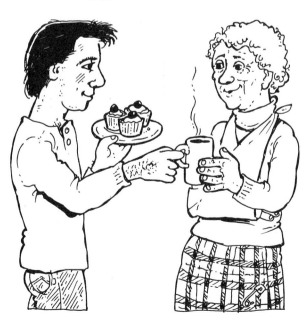

6 To be interested

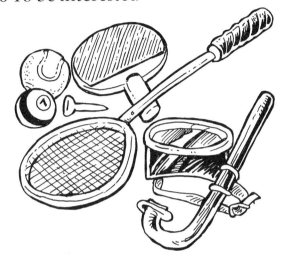

Well, you can get along with a boring job, a boring life, but very few human beings can live in solitary confinement or in complete silent darkness, as scientists have shown.

Bored people do all sorts of things, from getting pregnant to vandalism, from taking drugs to murder.

The simplest cure for teenage boredom is music.

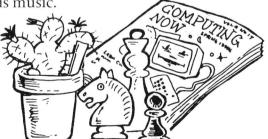

But some people need some of these more than others.

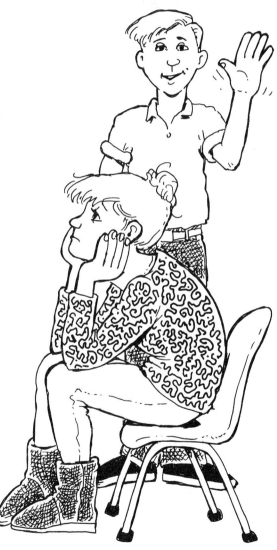

Maturity

NEEDS FULFILLED	As a child	As an adolescent	As a young adult	In middle-age	In old-age
Physical security	Provided by parents	Some provided by parents, some by yourself	You are responsible for rates, taxes, etc. Who wants to grow up?	Well, you've either got it by now or you'll never have it. Body begins to wear out	Provided by the Welfare State at least, probably your own pension as well
Respected by others	Mum matters most	Mum matters less now, Dad also important, and teachers. Friends matter more	Not too worried about others, except where cash and jobs are concerned	May be a bit bothered about what people say about your kids!	You don't have to worry about this. You can stay unwashed for as long as you like!
Respected by yourself	If Mum loves you, you love yourself	Shaky – you have to get a secure self-image by getting to know your new self	You are fairly secure at this age, but sometimes get savage knocks, e.g. from parents or parents-in-law	Very worrying. Have you succeeded in life? Are you starting to look old?	Too late to change now. If you respect yourself you'll get serenity if not wisdom!
To mate		Matters a lot to boys, not so urgent for girls	Problem is all the others you fancy!	Can get a bit boring – look for a new mate, new mating practices	Not so urgent. Some stop and are glad, some are sad for lost joys
To care for others		Matters more to girls, but there are some very caring boys about	You've got plenty to care for at this time of life	Especially for Mum, when all the kids are gone there is a big gap in her life. No-one to care for	Grandchildren – all the fun and none of the hard work
To be interested	Just give me lots of attention	Very important – everything can seem boring at this age	You are so busy, you've no time to be bored	You're so used to being busy, you need to take up new interests. A new job?	These who stay interested live longest and are happiest

Choosing your style

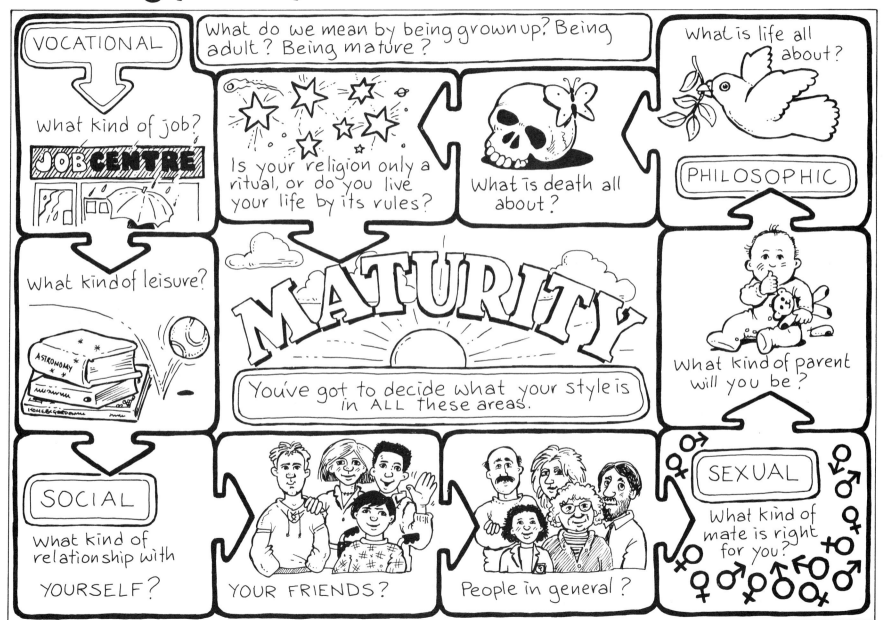

Ageing

When do we start to age?
It's a lifelong process.

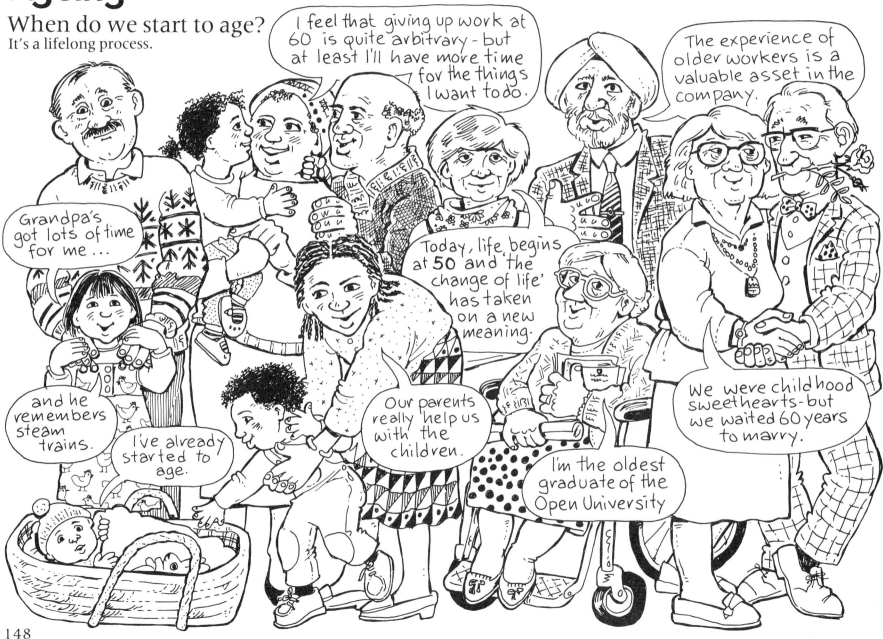

Physical changes and changing needs

My eyesight's not so good – hearing and smell too...

You need new spectacles.

I don't have such a big appetite – but then I can't eat everything I used to.

Come and have lunch with us at the day centre.

I worry about having an accident because cuts and fractures can take so long to heal.

I'll come round and make sure you've no loose rugs to slip on.

Although I don't feel the cold much, it's hard to keep warm.

I'll also make sure it's warm enough for you at home. You must not be a victim of HYPOTHERMIA.

I'm getting grey and wrinkled...

and I'm getting shorter.

Sometimes I'm a bit forgetful or uncertain about things.

You need more company and mental stimulation.

Road accidents and age

Teenage motorcyclists have a high accident rate.

Although reactions slow down with age, deaths in car accidents decrease up to the age of 50.

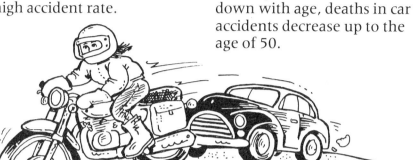

Is your mum menopausal?

The **menopause** happens to women in their late 40s.

The ovaries produce less of the hormone **oestrogen**.

Less oestrogen means:
1. no more plumpness due to water retention
2. hair and skin change and become drier, and may react differently to cosmetics
3. breasts and tummy lose firmness

Changes to blood vessels can mean:
1. cold sweats and hot flushes
2. swollen feet and legs
3. rapid heart beats

Changes in metabolism can lead to increase in weight.

The end of a woman's reproductive life can be a relief or a sadness – it depends on your point of view and your circumstances.

Do men have a menopause?

Their hormone levels drop gradually from age 17 onwards.

Hormones apart, in mid-life men and women can help each other to take stock of their lives and look forward to the years to come.

149

Death and life

How long a life can we expect?

In the Bible people lived to 'three score years and ten'. Today the average is still 70. Did people in the past really live to this age?

Iron Age   **Middle Ages**   **Mid 19th Century**

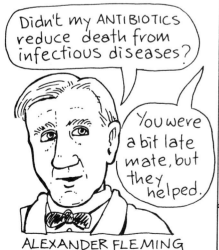

I died at 18

I died at 33

I died at 40

Our life expectancy changes according to how old we are.

At birth A boy can hope to live to 68.5 years.

At 20 A young man might expect to reach 70.6 years

At 50 It's increased even more to 72.7 years.

At 65 It's 76.9 years.

At 70 It's 79.3 years.

At 80 It's 85.4 years.

But death catches up eventually.
The longer you live the better chance of survival you have.

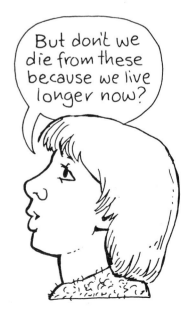

What do we die of today?

These changes are due to differences in lifestyles and the environment.

Didn't my ANTIBIOTICS reduce death from infectious diseases?

You were a bit late mate, but they helped.

ALEXANDER FLEMING

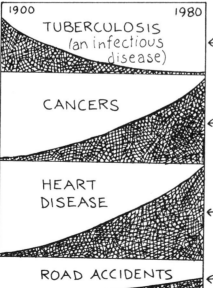

Deaths due to:

1900 ——— 1980

TUBERCULOSIS (an infectious disease)

CANCERS

HEART DISEASE

ROAD ACCIDENTS

← Fall due to better-fed people living in a healthier environment.

← Many cancers are believed to be caused by the environment and perhaps triggered by stress.

← Stress, diet, smoking and lack of exercise all contribute to deaths from heart disease.

← Road accidents increased as car ownership became more widespread.

But don't we die from these because we live longer now?

150

The ageing population

The proportion of old people in the population is increasing.

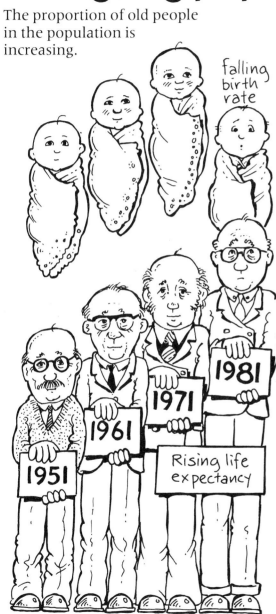

falling birth rate

Rising life expectancy

1951 1961 1971 1981

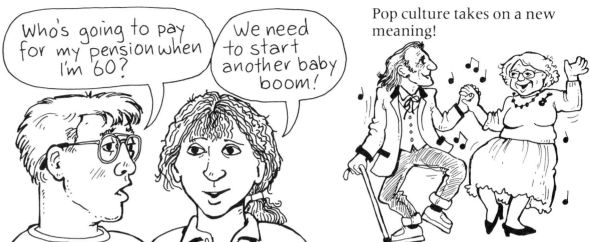

Who's going to pay for my pension when I'm 60?

We need to start another baby boom!

Pop culture takes on a new meaning!

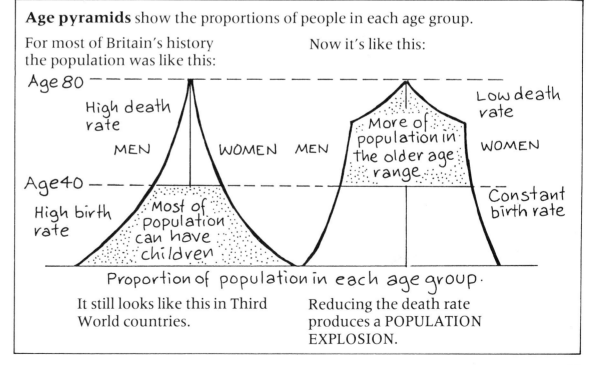

Age pyramids show the proportions of people in each age group.

For most of Britain's history the population was like this:

Now it's like this:

Age 80

High death rate

Low death rate

MEN   WOMEN   MEN

More of population in the older age range

WOMEN

Age 40

High birth rate

Most of population can have children

Constant birth rate

Proportion of population in each age group.

It still looks like this in Third World countries.

Reducing the death rate produces a POPULATION EXPLOSION.

Check-up 10 What do you know about how you grow and develop?

1 Say whether the following sentences are true or false?

(a) Genes are carried on chromosomes.
(b) Genes control the development of eye colour.
(c) Each cell in the body contains 56 chromosomes.
(d) An egg cell contains 23 chromosomes.
(e) Two brown-eyed parents cannot have a blue-eyed child.
(f) Two blue-eyed parents cannot have a brown-eyed child.
(g) Identical twins must always be the same sex.
(h) All human beings need to be respected by others.
(i) The menopause happens to women in their late 40s.
(j) In the 1990s there will be a higher proportion of young people in the British population than now.

2 Complete the graph to show how our life expectancy changes according to how old we are. Use the figures from page 150.

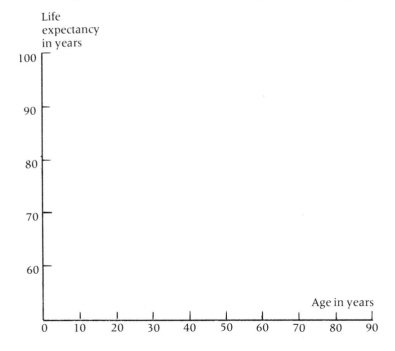

3 If you look at people around you, you can see that there is no such thing as 'normal'. People are different in many ways. To show these differences, carry out this survey of your friends and classmates.
Your survey should be in the form of a table like this.

Name	Age	Male/Female	Height	Shoe size	Weight	Eye colour	Hair colour

After carrying out your survey, answer the following questions.

(a) What is the height of the tallest person in your survey?
(b) What is the height of the shortest person in your survey?
(c) Make your survey results for height into a bar chart. Use these axes:

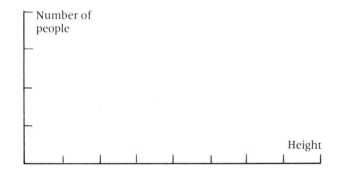

(d) What is the most common height of people in your survey?
(e) How many people did you have in your survey? Would your results have been very different if you had surveyed more people? Explain your answer.
(f) Do the tallest people also seem to be the heaviest?
(g) Do the tallest people seem to have the largest feet?
(h) Does a particular hair colour seem to go with a particular eye colour.

11 How You Reproduce

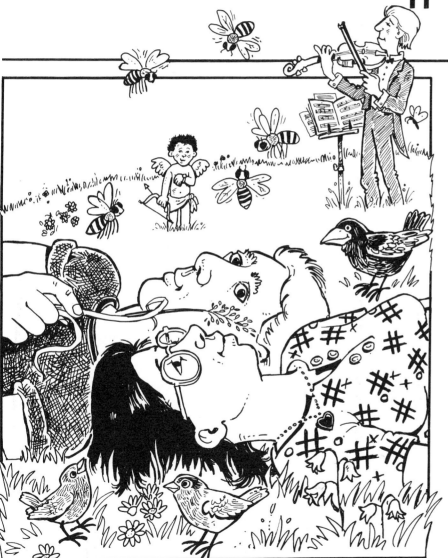

Sexual differences

At puberty our bodies begin to change quickly and the differences between boys and girls become more marked. In girls the **ovaries** mature and the production of eggs and menstruation start.

In boys the **testes** mature and the production of sperm and erections of the penis start.

BROADER SHOULDERS

BEARD

ARMPIT HAIR

BREASTS DEVELOP

BROADER HIPS

PUBIC HAIR

HAIR ON CHEST

LARGER PENIS AND TESTES

Changes in feelings and behaviour
These are affected by:
    how we see ourselves
    what society tells us.

Our sex is fixed at fertilization but these other sexual characteristics are affected by our sex hormones.

Female external sex organs:

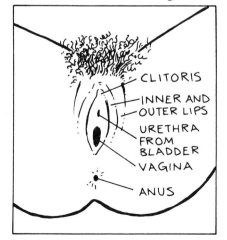

CLITORIS

INNER AND OUTER LIPS

URETHRA FROM BLADDER

VAGINA

ANUS

Other changes
In both boys and girls there is a growth spurt, and armpit and pubic hair grows. Boys start to grow a beard, get a deeper voice and become more muscular. In girls the hips become broader and breasts develop. Sex hormones produced by the ovaries and testes control development of these **secondary sexual characteristics**.

Male external sex organs:

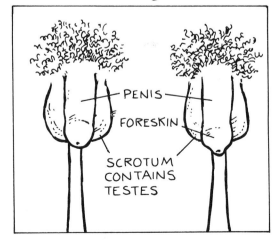

PENIS

FORESKIN

SCROTUM CONTAINS TESTES

Boys and girls worry about being normal adults

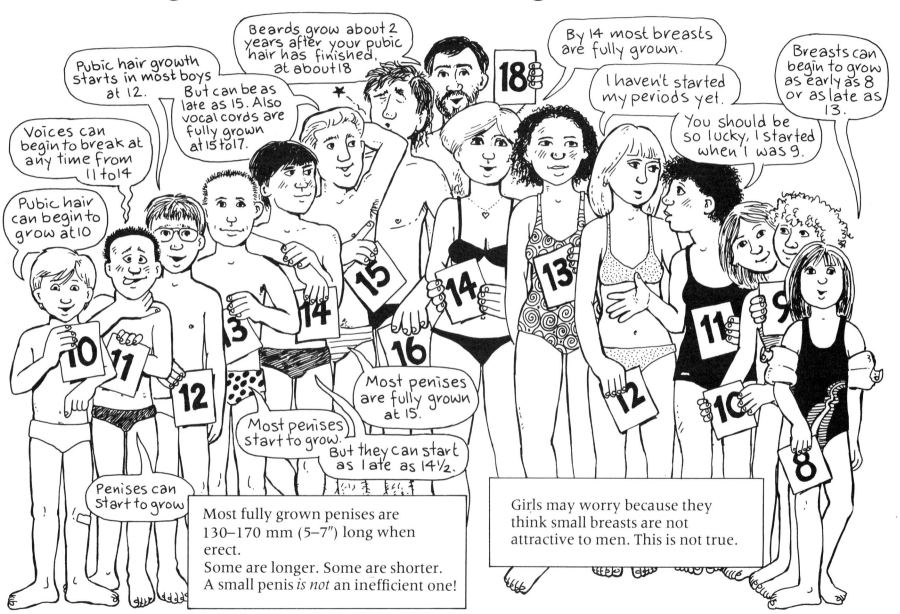

Hormones and behaviour – the menstrual cycle

Inside a woman there is a **uterus** or **womb**.
This is where a fertilized egg may grow into a baby.
The lining of the uterus is thick and soft with lots of blood to provide the baby with food and oxygen and to remove waste products.

This lining is changed for a new one every month:
● unless the woman becomes pregnant
● until she reaches the **menopause** at the age of about 50 when menstruation stops.

Every month women feel different at different times in the cycle. These feelings are due to **hormones**.
Hormones are chemicals produced by the **ovaries** under the influence of the brain.
Hormones act on the brain and make you feel and behave differently.

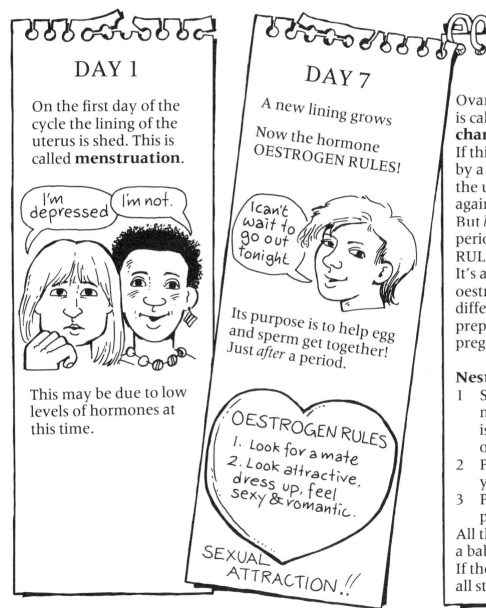

DAY 1

On the first day of the cycle the lining of the uterus is shed. This is called **menstruation**.

I'm depressed

I'm not.

This may be due to low levels of hormones at this time.

DAY 7

A new lining grows

Now the hormone OESTROGEN RULES!

I can't wait to go out tonight

Its purpose is to help egg and sperm get together! Just *after* a period.

OESTROGEN RULES
1. Look for a mate
2. Look attractive, dress up, feel sexy & romantic.

SEXUAL ATTRACTION..!!

DAY 14

Ovary sheds an egg. This is called **ovulation**. **All change**!
If this egg is not fertilized by a sperm, the lining of the uterus will be shed again.
But *before* the next period PROGESTERONE RULES!
It's a similar chemical to oestrogen but it has a different purpose, to prepare for a possible pregnancy.

Nest building
1   Stop looking for a mate: either the egg is fertilized by now or it is too old.
2   Protect yourself and your baby.
3   Prepare a nice clean place for the baby.
All this even if there isn't a baby.
If there isn't a baby this all starts again . . .

Your menstrual cycle

The menstrual cycle:
What sort of ride is yours?
Nobody's got a clockwork
uterus.

Are you the moody one? Up
and down all the time?
Do these changes of mood fit
in with your menstrual cycle?
They could be due to the
hormones **oestrogen** and
progesterone.

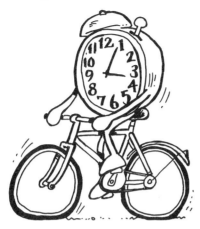

Women produce different
amounts of oestrogen and
progesterone

- at different times of life
- at different times of the
  year
- depending on how and
  where they live.

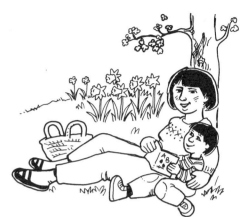

Physical feelings		Behaviour	
O	Feel great	P	Cry for no reason
O	Hair good, skin good	P	Can't concentrate
O	Stomach cramps	P	Anxious
O	Can't sleep	P	Tidy, urge to do jobs
P	Sweat more	P	Like staying in
P	Spotty, greasy skin	O	Like going out
△	Bra too small	O	Talkative
△	Put on weight	O	Feel good about self
△	Bruise easily	O	Feel romantic and
△	Can't pass water or		sexy
	can't stop		

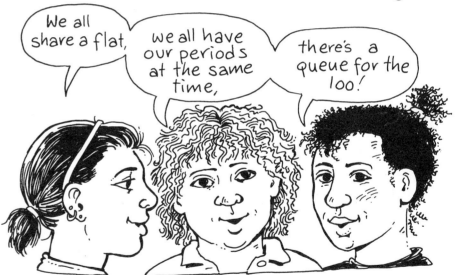

We all share a flat, we all have our periods at the same time, there's a queue for the loo!

O = due to oestrogen (or lack of it). Keeps water in body.

P = due to progesterone (or lack of it). Helps get rid of water.

△ = due to water retention, too much oestrogen or too little
    progesterone.

Everybody is different and hormones are only one influence
on how you behave.

So you can't blame your hormones every time you feel
miserable, yell at your mother, or fail your driving test.

Nature's gigantic plot

Most animals are at the mercy of 'Nature's gigantic plot': babies must be born at all costs so as to continue the species.

It's all part of **Nature's gigantic plot**!

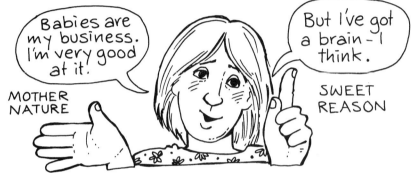

Babies are my business. I'm very good at it.

MOTHER NATURE

But I've got a brain – I think.

SWEET REASON

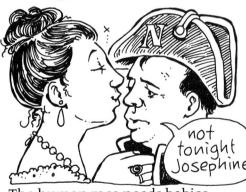

Men and women can think of lots of ways to avoid the pain and hard work that babies can mean.

not tonight Josephine.

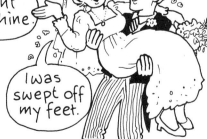

I was swept off my feet.

The human race needs babies to continue.
The human race survives because of hormones which can overcome logical thought!

158

Sexual attraction

How does it work? It's what you see.
Both boys and girls show they are attracted like this:

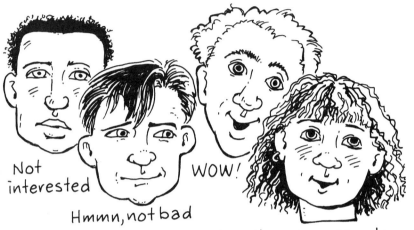

Not interested

Hmmn, not bad

WOW!

Eyes like this, signal back and attract the person who "WOW'ed you first.

What makes you say 'wow'?

You can stop yourself saying 'wow', but you can't stop your pupils dilating – try it.

Impulses go direct from your eyes to a gland which produces another hormone, **adrenalin**, which dilates your pupils.

Films, magazines, parents and friends have given you ideas or **stereotypes** of what is sexually attractive.

Attraction is also by smelling, touching, hearing and the person's personality.

Love, sex and chemistry

Don't ignore your hormones – get wise to them!

Girls

During a period   Don't think you are going mad, it's not you, just your hormones.

Just before a period   It's not a good time to take your driving test, but it is a good time to remember you don't always hate the ones you love.

After a period   Remember that your hormones are pushing you towards a mate. You could make dates for later in the month which you don't fancy when the time comes.

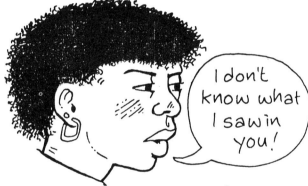

I don't know what I saw in you!

So at this time: tidy your room, get that dress finished. See page 149.

What else can you put on your list?
LOW HORMONE ACTIVITY OFTEN GIVES DEPRESSION:
1   Menstruation: just before, during or after
2   After an abortion or miscarriage (a natural abortion) Hormone treatment can help.
3   After you've had a baby   If it goes on for a long time or is very bad, see your doctor for some extra hormones.
4   During the menopause   Only 20% of women get hot flushes but everyone gets a hormone drop. See page 149.

Boys

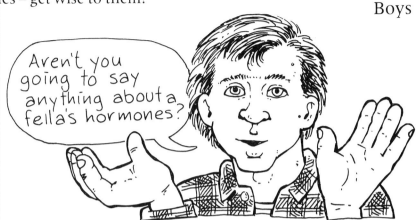

Aren't you going to say anything about a fella's hormones?

There's only one kind (not two).
It's called **testosterone**.
It makes you able to produce **sperm**.
It gives you all the signals to attract your mate and the drive to go out and find her.

It also gives you: acne, big muscles, and makes you go bald.

Your hormones are at a peak when you are between 17 and 23. After this your sex drive drops, but you can make up for it with experience.

So can't men blame middle age blues on a hormone drop? Yes – it starts at 17! But the drop is very gradual.
If the male menopause happens, it's probably less to do with low hormone levels than with other factors.

Final question
How can you tell the difference between LOVE and SEX (or Nature's gigantic plot)?

Conception

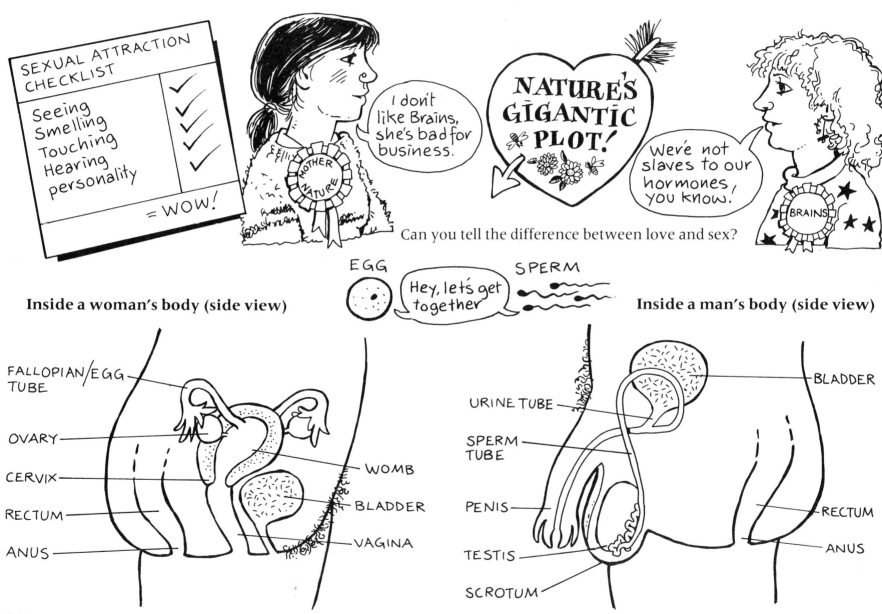

Can you tell the difference between love and sex?

Inside a woman's body (side view)

Inside a man's body (side view)

Our bodies are perfectly designed to allow millions of sperm to pass from the man to the egg inside the woman's body.

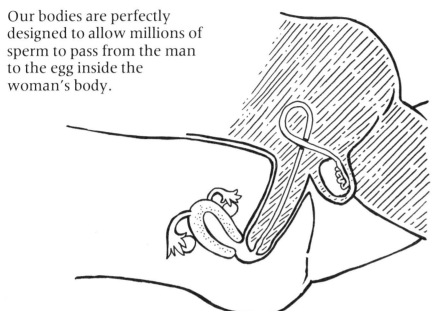

Sexual excitement makes the penis erect.

Sexual excitement makes the vagina slippery.

This excitement climaxes with millions of sperm in a white fluid (**semen**) shooting out of the man's penis into the woman's vagina.
The egg meets one sperm.

Fertilization can lead to this:

Sexually-transmitted diseases
AIDS is a very dangerous disease caused by a virus. The virus can destroy your body defences. You then catch all the infections going and you are also more likely to get cancer. People who have the AIDS virus usually die because of it. AIDS is passed from one person to another during sexual intercourse. At present there is no cure for AIDS.

Other diseases passed on during sexual intercourse are **syphilis** and **gonorrhoea**, which are caused by bacteria, and **genital herpes**, which is caused by a virus. Syphilis is particularly dangerous as it can damage the nervous system. Both syphilis and gonorrhoea can be treated successfully with antibiotics if diagnosed early. Herpes, like AIDS, has no cure, but although its effects are unpleasant (similar to cold sores) it is not fatal.

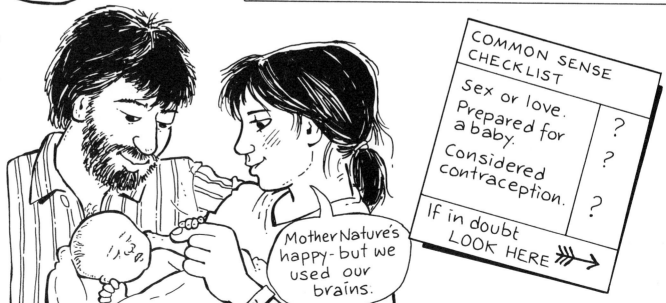

Mother Nature's happy - but we used our brains.

COMMON SENSE CHECKLIST

Sex or love. Prepared for a baby.	?
	?
Considered contraception.	?
If in doubt LOOK HERE ⇒	

161

Contraception: who wants a baby?

Did they know the difference between love and sex?

In love with her?
Try changing the word *love* for *sex* in songs, stories, what people say.

Do you only go with him/her because you like being seen with him/her because he/she is so gorgeous to look at?

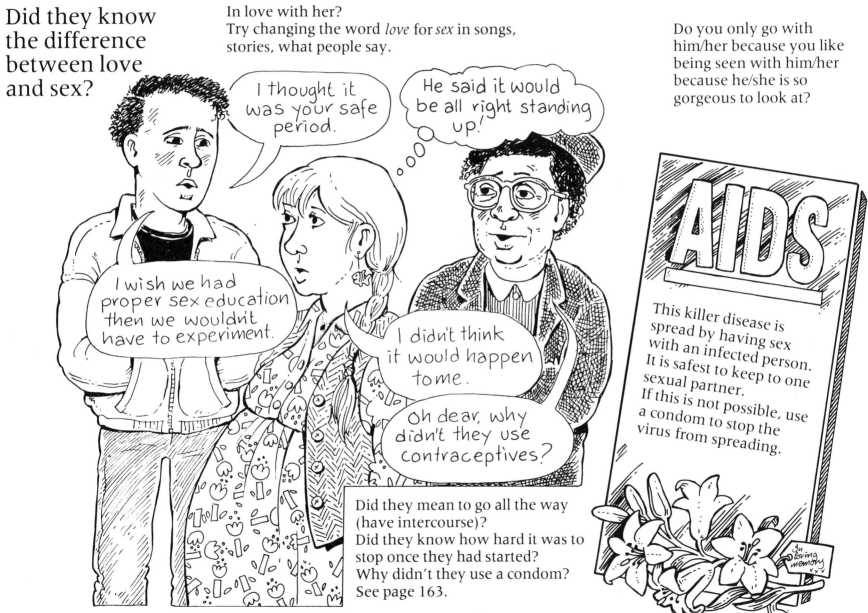

I thought it was your safe period.

He said it would be all right standing up!

I wish we had proper sex education then we wouldn't have to experiment.

I didn't think it would happen to me.

Oh dear, why didn't they use contraceptives?

Did they mean to go all the way (have intercourse)?
Did they know how hard it was to stop once they had started?
Why didn't they use a condom?
See page 163.

AIDS

This killer disease is spread by having sex with an infected person.
It is safest to keep to one sexual partner.
If this is not possible, use a condom to stop the virus from spreading.

In loving memory
xxx

Family planning – for planned families

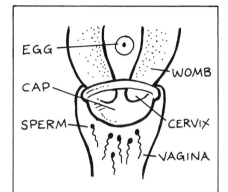

A cap/diaphragm fits over the cervix at the end of the womb and stops sperm getting through the cervix into the womb.

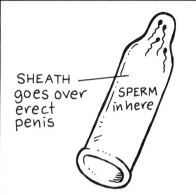

A sheath/condom/durex keeps sperm from getting to the egg.

Both work better with a spermicide jelly to kill the sperm.

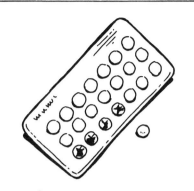

Oral contraceptive pills contain hormones which stop the ovaries producing an egg every month – if you remember to take them!

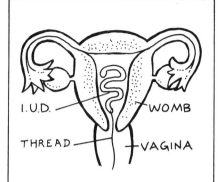

A loop/coil/IUD inserted in the womb prevents a fertilized egg developing any further.

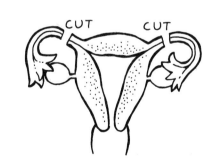

Sterilization: by cutting the egg tubes and sealing the ends.

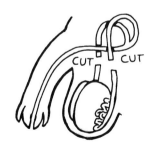

In men the sperm tubes are cut and sealed in a **vasectomy**.

Did they want a dream baby?

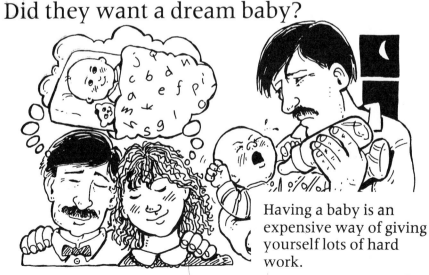

Having a baby is an expensive way of giving yourself lots of hard work.

Pregnancy

Signs of pregnancy

1 Periods cease

2 Morning sickness

3 Increase in weight

4 Breasts swell and nipples darken

5 Abdomen gets bigger (stretch marks)

6 Bigger uterus puts pressure on the bladder and diaphragm.

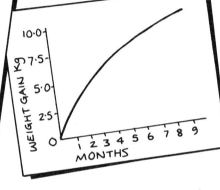

ANTENATAL TESTS
during pregnancy
NAME: Ms D. Dallas.
- ✓ General health.
- ✓ Weight.
- ✓ Lungs and heart.
- ✓ Blood.
  - Group e.g. Rhesus Neg.
  - Iron deficiency.
  - Sexually transmitted disease.
  - Pressure.
- ✓ Urine
  - To confirm pregnancy (presence of hormones).
  - Test for toxaemia.
- ✓ Progress & Position of baby.
- ✓ Size of Pelvis.
- ✓ Cervical smear test for cancer of the womb

Weight goes up by some 10 kg but baby only weighs 3–3.5 kg. What's the rest? (See page 165.)

WEIGHT GAIN Kg — 10.0, 7.5, 5.0, 2.5, 0 — 1 2 3 4 5 6 7 8 9 MONTHS

Egg meets sperm

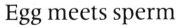

FERTILIZATION.

24 HOURS fertilized egg divides into two.

48 HOURS 4 cells.

3 DAYS 8 cells.

4 DAYS EMBRYO of 32 cells.

On the fifth day the embryo reaches the womb and buries itself in the lining.
If something is wrong, natural miscarriage may occur.

The baby

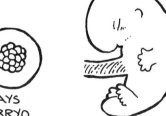

AT ONE MONTH i've got; a brain and heart, eyes, ears, mouth, tiny arms and legs, a tail and am 6mm.

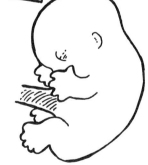

AT TWO MONTHS i'm a FOETUS, but i'm still only 25mm long, that's 10,000 × bigger than the egg.

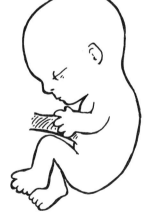

THREE MONTHS.

164

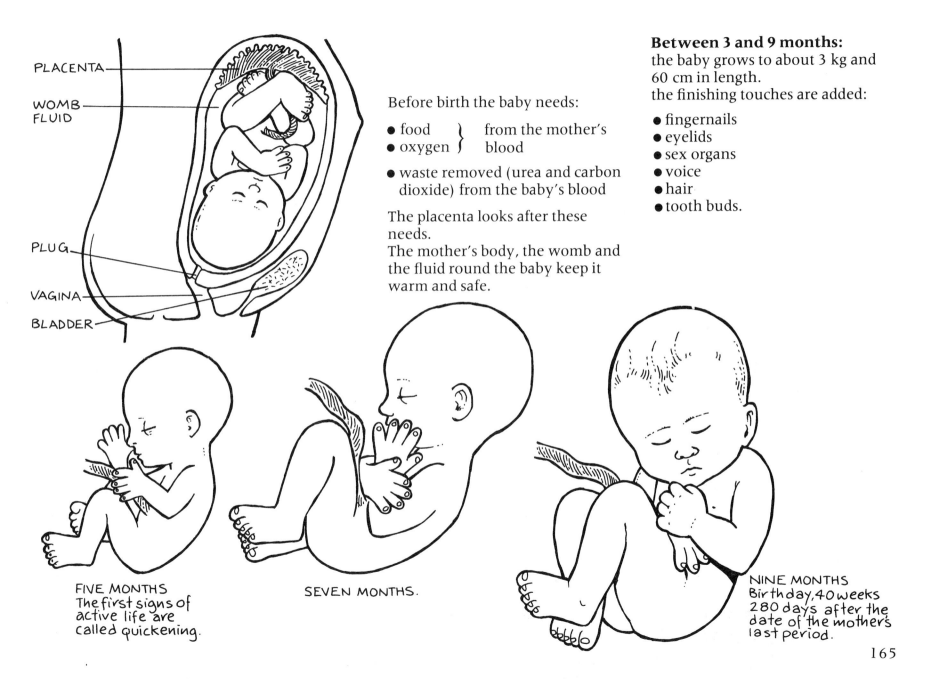

PLACENTA

WOMB FLUID

PLUG

VAGINA

BLADDER

Before birth the baby needs:

- food ⎫ from the mother's
- oxygen ⎭ blood

- waste removed (urea and carbon dioxide) from the baby's blood

The placenta looks after these needs.
The mother's body, the womb and the fluid round the baby keep it warm and safe.

Between 3 and 9 months:
the baby grows to about 3 kg and 60 cm in length.
the finishing touches are added:

- fingernails
- eyelids
- sex organs
- voice
- hair
- tooth buds.

FIVE MONTHS
The first signs of active life are called quickening.

SEVEN MONTHS.

NINE MONTHS
Birthday, 40 weeks 280 days after the date of the mother's last period.

165

Birth

GET READY . . . GET SET . . . GO!
The baby settles down in the womb
ready for birth.

First stage of labour
The neck of the womb (cervix) opens
up around the baby's head.

Second stage of labour
The baby is born.

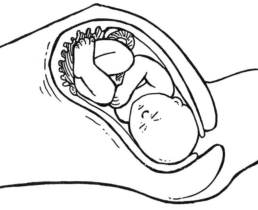

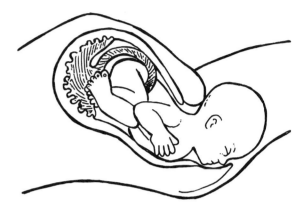

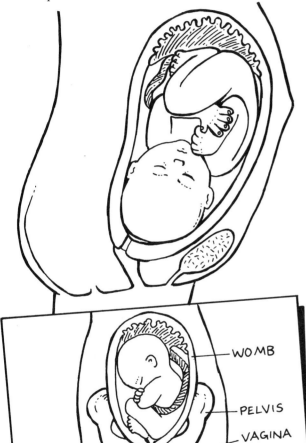

The plug in the opening to the womb
comes out (the 'show').
The muscles in the womb start to
contract and push the baby out.
The bag round the baby breaks and the
water comes out.

WOMB

PELVIS

VAGINA

Sometimes the baby gets it wrong
and sits like this . . . not like this
This is a breech birth position.

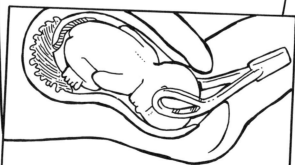

Even if it is the right way up, the
baby sometimes needs extra help
and forceps may be used.

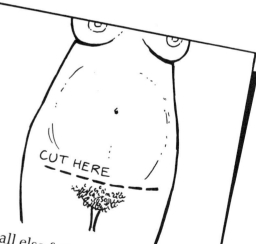

CUT HERE

If all else fails the baby can be
delivered by a Caesarian
operation.

Third stage of labour
The womb contracts and pushes out the **placenta** (afterbirth).

The newborn baby
The cord is cut and eventually drops off, leaving a scar – the baby's navel.

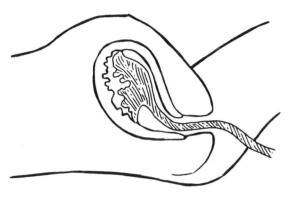

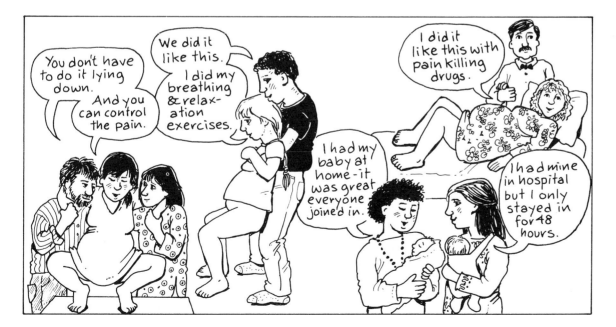

The new baby can:
● walk
● grasp
  (although these skills are quickly lost)
● suck milk from breast or bottle
● breathe air using its lungs.

The new baby needs:
● food
● air
● warmth
● security
● protection
● love.

What do you think birth is like from the baby's point of view?

Check-up 11 What do you know about how you reproduce?

1   Here is a list of changes that take place during puberty.
Make a table like the one shown below. Put each change in the
correct column in the table. Some changes may fit into both
columns.

Muscles become bigger
Sperms start to be made
Hair grows on chest
Breasts develop
Hair grows under arms
Periods begin

Voice becomes deeper
Egg cells start to be released
   from ovaries
Hair grows on face
Penis becomes larger
Pubic hair grows

Changes in girls at puberty	Changes in boys at puberty

2   Say whether the following sentences are true or false.

   (a)   All girls start their periods by the time they are 13.
   (b)   The male sex hormone is called testosterone.
   (c)   All boys stop growing when they are 16.
   (d)   Identical twins are formed from an egg which has joined
         with one sperm.
   (e)   All boys have bigger muscles than all girls.
   (f)   There is no such thing as the male menopause.
   (g)   All penises are between 5 and 7 inches long when erect.
   (h)   Having sex while standing up is a good form of
         contraception.
   (i)   Girls shouldn't go swimming during their period.
   (j)   A two-month-old foetus is approximately 25 cm in length.

3   (a)   Make a drawing of the female reproductive organs like the
         one below. Label the following on your drawing.

   ovary   uterus   cervix   vagina   fallopian tubes

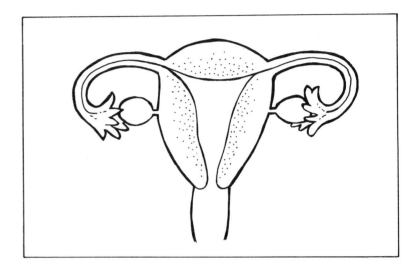

   (b)   Mark on the drawing the route taken
         (i) by an ovum when it is released from an ovary.
         (ii) by a sperm entering the womb.
   (c)   Show where fertilization is likely to happen.
   (d)   Mark a possible place where the fertilized egg may begin to
         develop.
   (e)   How many days after an egg is fertilized does it bury itself in
         the womb wall?
   (f)   Name a contraceptive which can stop the sperm from
         getting into the womb.
   (g)   Name a contraceptive which can stop the fertilized egg from
         developing inside the womb.
   (h)   Write a sentence to explain how the pill stops a baby from
         being produced.
   (i)   Which part of the baby should leave the womb first during
         birth?

168

12 Diagnosis and Cures

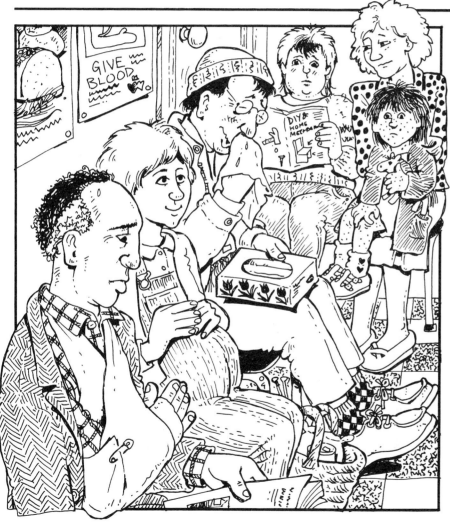

Diagnosis is for doctors
When to see your doctor
But doctors say such different things!
What's causing your headache?
Check-up 12

Diagnosis is for doctors

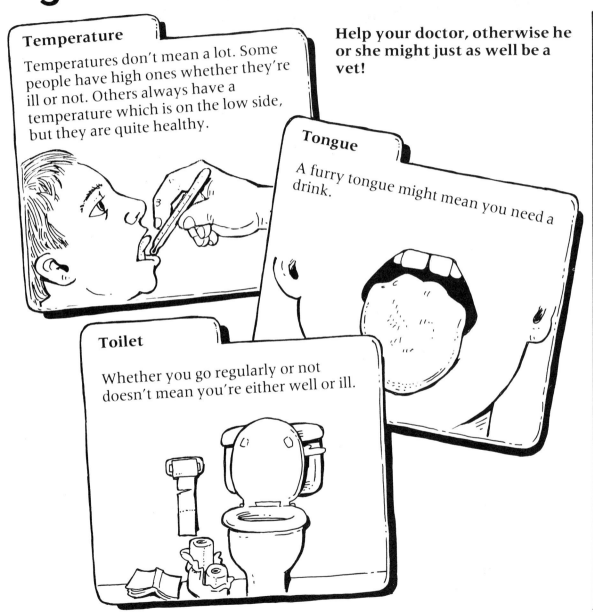

Temperature

Temperatures don't mean a lot. Some people have high ones whether they're ill or not. Others always have a temperature which is on the low side, but they are quite healthy.

Tongue

A furry tongue might mean you need a drink.

Toilet

Whether you go regularly or not doesn't mean you're either well or ill.

Help your doctor, otherwise he or she might just as well be a vet!

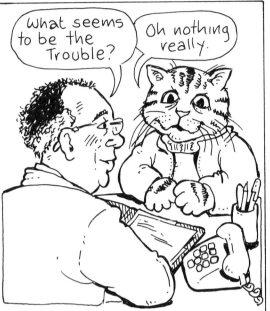

What seems to be the Trouble?

Oh nothing really.

1 Talk to your doctor, don't wait for him/her to ask all the questions.

2 Write what you want to say down before you see your doctor. Often what you are really worried about seems so silly when you get there that you don't mention it – until you're leaving. This wastes the doctor's time and yours.

3 You don't have to be covered with purple spots to be ill. If you're worried see your doctor.

When to see your doctor

Backache
To avoid backache
- Lift things properly (see page 107).
- Put a board (e.g. an old door) under your mattress. If you are buying a new mattress choose a firm one.
- Try heat – hot water bottle, electric blanket, warmer clothes, and no gap between jeans and sweater.

If you still have a backache after two weeks **S**ee **Y**our **D**octor (SYD).

Burns bigger than a 5p piece?
SYD

Coughing   Chemists have some good cures. If you have tried them for more than three weeks –
SYD

Colds and flu   Bed, hot drinks, vitamin C and paracetamol are more use than doctors! And when everyone's got flu, people with weak chests need the doctor most.

Depression often follows flu. But if you have lots of depression and no flu, SYD. It's a real illness and can be cured.

Dizziness   Girls may feel dizzy before menstruation (periods).
SYD

Lack of sleep or too much alcohol can also make you dizzy. But if you have deafness, ear pain, ringing noises in your head or if the dizziness persists –
SYD

Ears   Wax in your ears, pain, discharge and even just crackle –
Don't fiddle with them yourself.
SYD

Joints   If they are painful or swollen –
SYD

Mouth ulcers   Get pain-killing lozenges from a chemist. If you keep getting them it may be a sign that you are run down –
SYD

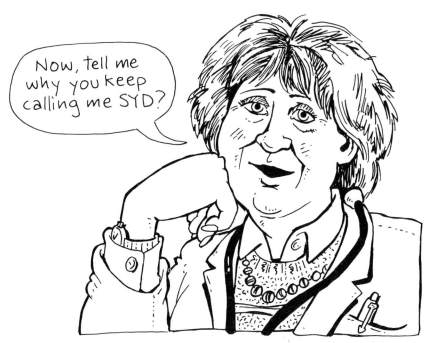

But doctors say such different things

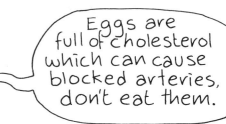

ALL HUMAN BEINGS ARE DIFFERENT THROUGH HEREDITY AND IN THEIR HABITS

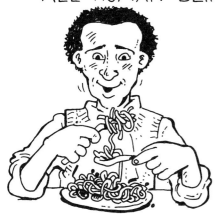

Some can eat bread, cakes and chips and never get fat. Others just have to look at a cream cake – in your mouth for half a minute, round your hips for the rest of your life.

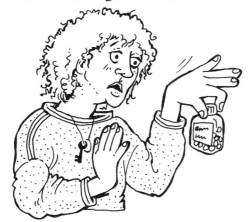

Some are poisoned by penicillin. Most people are made well by it.

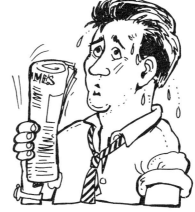

Some people are always warm; some are too warm! Others 'feel the cold' and never go on winter sports holidays.

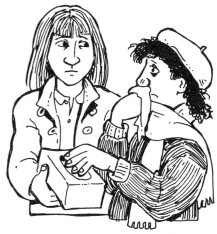

Some never catch colds and flu. Others are never without a damp nose and a wheeze.

SO FIND OUT WHAT SUITS YOU AND WHAT IS CAUSING YOUR PROBLEMS.

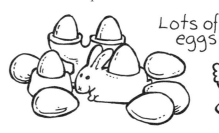

Lots of eggs?

A few eggs?

No eggs?

What is causing your headache?

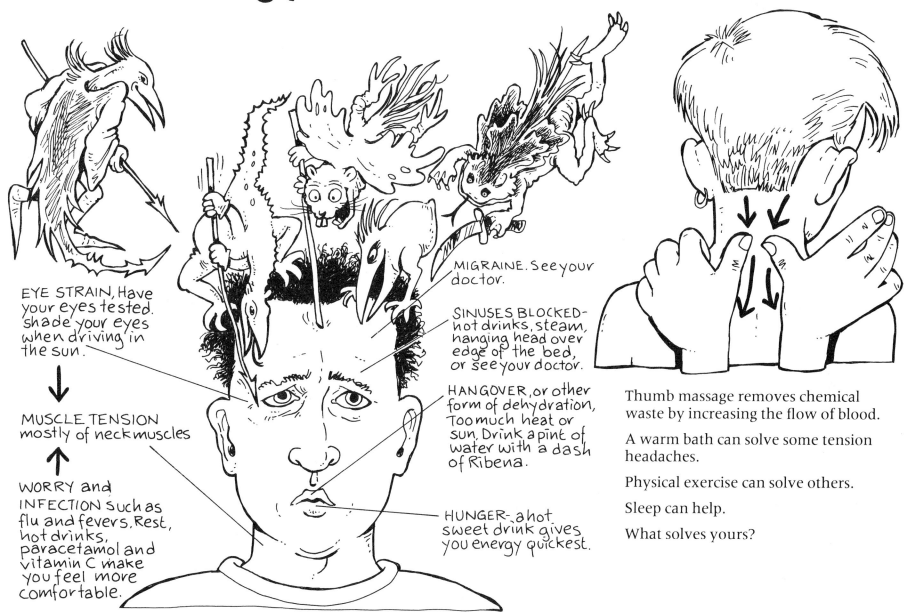

EYE STRAIN, Have your eyes tested. Shade your eyes when driving in the sun.

MUSCLE TENSION mostly of neck muscles

WORRY and INFECTION such as flu and fevers. Rest, hot drinks, paracetamol and vitamin C make you feel more comfortable.

MIGRAINE. See your doctor.

SINUSES BLOCKED - hot drinks, steam, hanging head over edge of the bed, or see your doctor.

HANGOVER, or other form of dehydration, Too much heat or sun, Drink a pint of water with a dash of Ribena.

HUNGER - a hot sweet drink gives you energy quickest.

Thumb massage removes chemical waste by increasing the flow of blood.

A warm bath can solve some tension headaches.

Physical exercise can solve others.

Sleep can help.

What solves yours?

173

Check-up 12 What do you know about diagnosis and cures?

1   Look at these different ways of keeping healthy or curing illness.

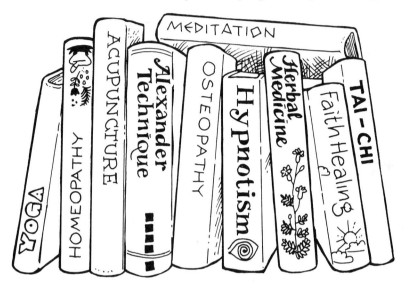

Find out something about each method. Ask other people what they know about them.

2   In this word search there are ten symptoms of illness. Write down each symptom and say whether you would need to see a doctor if you had this symptom.

```
Z H T B L K J D W Q
D E P R E S S I O N
C A J I X O L Z V E
L D B W R Y Y Z P C
D A A N P B T Y M I
H C C I A K M L U J
Y H K T I R E D O Q
D E A F N E S S Y X
L X C O U G H I J C
G Z H I W L L C P E
K F E V E R M K V R
```

Index

Photographic Acknowledgements

Barnaby's Picture Library, 79, 111, 116 *(right)*
Biophoto Associates, 23, 41, 53, 98 *(top and bottom)* 99, 105, 141
British Coal, 9
Camera Press Ltd, 95, 103, 107
Sally & Richard Greenhill, 116 *(centre)*, 131 *(right)*
Indusphoto, 9
Ivor Leonard/The Spastics Society, 131 *(centre)*
Mencap, 131 *(left)*
St. Bartholomew's Hospital, 112 *(right)*
Science Photo Library, 47, 48, 52, 106
Topham, 112 *(left)*, 116 *(left)*